To Michael, my Sunshine. I thoug
the darkness – you were the light i
the tunnel and you gui

To Ross, my rock. You never gave up on me and I will spend the rest of our lives making you glad that you stayed.

Alcohol……..

I drank for happiness and became unhappy
I drank for joy and became miserable
I drank for sociability and became argumentative
I drank for sophistication and became obnoxious
I drank for friendship and made enemies
I drank for sleep and woke tired
I drank for strength and felt weak
I drank for relaxation and got the shakes
I drank for courage and became afraid
I drank for confidence and became doubtful
I drank to make conversation easier and slurred my speech
I drank to feel heavenly and ended up feeling like hell

Anonymous

Introduction

There are many books available which address alcoholism, getting sober, and the challenges faced by those who have managed to achieve sobriety as they negotiate life's complications and raw emotions without the help of a drink to make it all go away. I have probably read most of them over the years, during my many desperate attempts to get– and stay– sober. Active alcoholism is a very scary and desperately lonely place. Reading anything about alcoholism and recovery, looking for the answer to the question 'why me' and attempting to make sense of it, (for example, endlessly 'Googling' famous people who have beaten alcoholism and reading their stories), fleetingly provided me with a sense of comfort and hope.

But what if, like me, you find yourself a hopeless alcoholic at the bottom of a downward spiral, now totally defeated and unable to stop drinking after going through all of the well-documented phases of alcoholism and the various tried and tested ways to beat it? Ill, terrified and alone.

I have not found a book written by someone who came back from that.

The brutal fact is that most people do die prematurely if they reach the point where they simply cannot live without a drink, because when your day to day existence is in the total grip of alcohol, there is very little hope of pulling back from it.

There are many people like I was, who have reached that heart-breaking realisation that they have failed to 'conquer' their alcoholism and to remain sober after attempts at rehab, AA meetings, SMART Recovery, Counselling - the list goes on. I know the overwhelming feelings of guilt, shame and fear that consume you when you have had your last ditch attempt at AA or rehab and started drinking again, throwing away in a couple of seconds the trust and hope of those who love you, that took many months to earn. I still vividly remember how absolutely gut-wrenching it is to run out of options and actually begin to accept that you are going to die from something that started as such a blast; something which at first seemed so innocent and normal.

For those people in the absolute depths of despair, feeling scared and alone, I have written this book. Reading this, I want you to imagine me holding your hand, looking you in the eye, and telling you to never give up hope, because I was where you are now.

You may be reading this book having not reached that stage yet. Perhaps you or your loved ones may be worried about your drinking, or you may have been to the GP about your alcohol consumption, had counselling, been to AA meetings, or even spent time in rehab. No matter how far down the alcoholic spiral you are, the fact that you are reading this book suggests that you have concerns about your drinking.

For those people, believe me, everything that you have read or have been told about alcoholism is true. It is progressive, merciless, and ultimately wants to kill you.

I make no apologies for being so blunt, because alcohol almost killed me and I was gradually losing everyone I love and everything dear to me, even though I had also been so sure that this could never happen to me. This book may also be useful for those who know or love an alcoholic and are struggling to understand why they continue to drink, even when their life has fallen apart or they are in a physical decline because of their drinking – I understand how helpless you feel.

At this point I should also stress that the purpose of this book is not to unfairly criticise AA (Alcoholics Anonymous), rehab, counselling, SMART therapy and any of the other treatments I have tried over the years. I know that these approaches do help some alcoholics and have saved people from drinking themselves to death. I am also eternally grateful to the many people I met over the years through AA and in the rehabs I attended, because they have all contributed in some way to who I am now. Ultimately, however, these approaches did not work for me and they don't work for many people. What I want to do is challenge the notion that if these paths don't lead to sobriety, it's because the alcoholic didn't try hard enough or because they didn't want to get sober.

The reality is that although AA and rehab are still the 'go to' options for most alcoholics and their GP's, friends and families, they simply don't work for many people. I appreciate that this may seem a controversial and provocative thing to say, but I believe that the fact that they are still put on a pedestal despite an almost complete lack of accountability or any meaningful success rate statistics needs to be talked about. I believe my personal experience is evidence of this.

We are all aware of high profile alcoholics who enter rehab multiple times after relapsing, sometimes after a long period of sobriety. This is also happening to countless ordinary alcoholics all of the time, the difference being that most ordinary alcoholics cannot afford to keep going back.

For those close to an alcoholic, this is an important topic, because they often find themselves at their wits end when an expensive stint in rehab has failed or they find out that a loved one has continued to drink whilst attending AA. It is so difficult for the friends and relatives of an alcoholic who starts to drink again after a period of abstinence, and it is completely understandable that they cannot comprehend why this happens, watching helplessly as their friend or loved one tries to get well and wants to get well, but their life continues to fall apart as they drink.

AA and rehab are still the most obvious 'solutions' that spring to mind when trying to get help for someone with a drinking problem, but when they don't work an alcoholic can find it difficult to explain why, because of feelings of shame and guilt about wasted money and also because they feel that they have let everyone down. Those around them can be forgiven for assuming that they just didn't try hard enough, or that they just don't want to stop drinking and I think that my experiences provide a useful illustration of why this is not necessarily the case.

I am not making excuses for alcoholics or portraying people who end up like I was as victims, I am simply using my own personal journey down the alcoholic spiral to try to explain what it's like - and I do not come out of this looking particularly good, but this book is not a vanity project and I have written it in an honest attempt to offer help and hope.

The book is also not a guide as to why people become alcoholics or, for that matter, why I think I became an alcoholic. There are so many reasons and underlying factors and every alcoholic is an individual who has their own story. In contrast, the story of alcoholism is depressingly predictable and, once you are in its grip, the stories may differ in terms of the characters and geography, but they follow a familiar beginning, middle and end. Sadly, the story of an active alcoholic who does not conquer their addiction to alcohol only has one ending.

Whether you believe that alcoholism is a disease, regard it as an unlucky outcome of liking a drink a bit too much, a physical addiction or just weakness is also, to me, irrelevant. Who cares about definitions when you are lying alone in bed, sobbing and praying whilst throwing up into a towel next to you, too ill and shaky to make it to the toilet or even lift your head? Who cares about definitions when you feel so alone even when you are with people, because your life has become one big lie and you are ashamed of the secret existence that you find yourself in, lying in bed frozen with fear because withdrawal from alcohol is causing you to hallucinate and see 'real' spiders swarming over your bed covers?

I need to write this book because I know how it feels to realise that you truly are at the end of the road, but drinking alcohol still seems to make sense - your only comfort. I have been so 'insane' and demented, that a life living totally on my own without anyone at all to interfere with my drinking seemed somehow appealing, (my son, my husband, my friends, my family, had gradually become less important to me than drinking alcohol).

Being awake was to drink and drinking was to pass out. Waking up at three in the morning and drinking to oblivion seemed completely normal. In recent years I had woken up in hospital, not remembering how I had gotten there, had run-ins with the police, hurt and lied to everyone I loved, embarrassed myself and those who cared about me, looked and felt increasingly ill and dishevelled and didn't care about my personal hygiene.

I was dying and I knew it and I was so completely heartbroken and frightened that it had come to this but, at the same time, I was terrified at the prospect of not being able to drink. I had tried everything to stop and had, on many occasions, managed sobriety for a period of time, (from a few weeks, to several months), but always, eventually started drinking again. This pathetic, tragic, sad and frightening life evolved from being just a normal, fun loving young woman who liked a drink and letting my hair down and continued to do so over my years as a career driven professional woman to a loving, stay at home mother.

Because of this I again make no apologies that this book is brutally honest about the realities of full blown alcoholism and not the sanitised version that you see in films. Where being covered in vomit and having horrendous stomach cramps and diarrhoea because of withdrawal, but not making it to the toilet isn't unusual, and where being stripped of every ounce of dignity and self-respect and the respect of everyone who knows you is where you now find yourself - all of this began with loving a drink.

But even though my journey is alarming and at times horrific, I have found true happiness and, more importantly, complete freedom. Freedom from alcohol, cravings, weekly meetings, temptation, shame….. freedom from a living hell.

So, if you are like I was at the end of my alcoholic existence, feeling hopeless and heartbroken and resigned to an early death because you have run out of options, but you still have some rare moments when you aren't comatose and you cry and beg someone or something to help, this is my way of holding your hand and telling you that there is still hope. You can still beat alcoholism and you can get the 'you' back that you have lost along the way, because I did - you should never give up.

I know what it is to reach the end of the line with alcoholism. I know what it felt like when I believed I would die very soon. Most people who reach that stage do not survive. They drink themselves to death.

I did survive.

Here is my story.

Chapter 1

Loving a Drink to Problem Drinking

I want to provide what may seem to be a quite 'matter of fact' account of how I progressed through the stages of alcoholism, a progression which I never thought could actually happen to me, because for a long time I genuinely believed that I was somehow immune to becoming an alcoholic. The next three chapters show how I gradually changed from simply being someone who liked a drink, to being a heavy drinker and then from being a heavy drinker to a problem drinker and then from being a problem drinker to a functioning alcoholic. Ultimately I became someone who just couldn't stop drinking and was in total despair and I resigned myself to the fact that I was going to die because of alcohol, (whether that be from an alcohol related illness, an accident, a car crash or taking my own life whilst intoxicated, which many alcoholics do).

My reason for being so matter of fact is simple – I want this book to help people like me. I do not want to write an entertaining account of my love affair with alcohol which turned into a nightmare and then had a happy ending of recovery, with chapter upon chapter of childhood memories and drinking stories. This is because I know that, if you are feeling like I was at the end, you most certainly will not be interested in reading the story of my life and you will not want to wade through someone else's embarrassing drinking stories – you will by now have plenty of your own. I want you to know that I understand that funny drinking anecdotes are a long distant memory for you and you are now living a life of fear, loneliness and pain, just as I was at the end. I also do not want to glamorise drinking and being drunk in any way – for an alcoholic, alcohol is nothing but a poisonous chemical.

I think it would be useful to use my experiences to illustrate how alcoholism is progressive for three different groups of people who might benefit from reading this book. First of all, for those people who really do feel that they have reached a point of no hope, I want you to know that I genuinely did get to the desperate place where you now find yourself. Secondly, for those people who know that they have a drink problem and are reading this book to either reassure themselves that they aren't an alcoholic or to work out if they are, you will definitely be able to identify where you are on the downward 'spiral' with reference to my story and to understand where you are potentially heading.

And finally, for the families and friends of alcoholics, I want to hopefully shed some light on the power that alcohol has over people, even when they so obviously want to stop drinking. I do know how heart-breaking and frustrating it is for you and how helpless you feel, but hopefully my experiences will help you to understand how apparent 'failure' to stop drinking may not be through lack of trying – I tried desperately hard to stay sober.

My need to write this book has also partly come from my frustration that the options available to alcoholics remain limited, predominantly, to AA, rehab and counselling. This has been the situation for years, even though many people, like me, find that these approaches don't work and they continue to drink until alcohol gradually robs them of everything dear to them.

In my own very simple terms, alcoholism can be divided into four stages: early, middle, late and then end stage. The harsh reality is that most people who reach end stage alcoholism die earlier than they should.

In the early stage, alcohol may be used in social situations to lessen anxiety and maybe 'loosen up', but because people become 'tolerant' to alcohol, they need larger amounts to get the same effect. This leads them to the middle stage when drinking increasing amounts of alcohol leads to the person embarrassing themselves and other negative consequences. However, they continue to drink regardless, needing more and more alcohol for the same effect, (because their tolerance levels continue to increase), eventually moving into late stage alcoholism, with more and more negative consequences, to the point where friends and family may express concerns. There will also most likely be health issues and accidents because of alcohol.

Eventually, the person may become an end stage alcoholic, when their whole life revolves around alcohol, their relationships, job and health suffer and they live to drink – a living hell until they die because of alcohol. At every stage of this process, alcohol convinces them that things will get better, they will be able to get back to normal drinking again and, most importantly, that they are not an alcoholic and anyone who says that they are is wrong.

It is scary how the progression of alcoholism can be so gradual that in the early years it often goes unnoticed, especially by those closest to an alcoholic. In those early years, something may happen when we have a drink that is mildly embarrassing, out of character or maybe even slightly upsetting, which sets a few alarm bells ringing, but is ultimately forgotten as life moves on.

Then life goes back to normal for a while, until another event occurs, perhaps more alarming than the last - a fall, a fight, harsh words etc. After apologies the next day and a period of shame, guilt and remorse, the embarrassment recedes and the cycle continues. Friends and loved ones may have niggling worries about the alcoholic, but they will often feel guilty about suspecting that someone has a drinking problem or they feel reluctant to broach the subject for fear of upsetting or insulting the person they care about.

What makes it even more difficult and confusing for those around an alcoholic is that even functioning alcoholics can still achieve great things and hold down jobs, (I invented a product and brought it to market during the years that my drinking progressed to the point where I became a functioning alcoholic). In the later years, however, it is alarming how rapidly things escalate and how the events fuelled by alcohol go from being mildly embarrassing or upsetting to perhaps dangerous or catastrophic, and how the periods of time in between these catastrophic events become smaller and smaller until, ultimately, alcohol is running the show completely and normal life disintegrates.

The combination of alcoholics being such convincing liars and their loved ones desperately wanting to believe what they are being told, means that alcohol stealthily and quietly settles into the life of the alcoholic and those around them, sometimes seemingly lying 'dormant', while it gathers its strength again. I have always imagined alcohol as the sinister dark shadows in the film Ghost, which creep out of the ground and slide towards their victim, enveloping them and ultimately dragging them to hell.

In the same way, my alcoholic personality gradually took over me, exaggerated by each glass of wine that I consumed – my own dark shadow. This dark shadow changed me from being a polite, caring and fun loving person into an aggressive, manipulative, selfish liar and this became more profound the more alcohol I consumed. It actually took years for my dark shadow to completely consume me, almost like a parasite, but even in the early years, the impact of alcohol on my personality was quite negative and it was happy to bide its time, creeping in and out of my life with increasing frequency as the years went by.

What I want to get across very clearly is the absolute power and control that alcohol has over an alcoholic in the end, after their journey down the spiral. It has made me feel so very ashamed re-visiting the awful lows that alcohol took me to and re-living the absolute chaos, hurt and devastation that I caused - especially to my son Michael, my husband Ross and my ex-husband Mark, but also to my family and friends, that I almost gave up on writing this book.

However, if by sharing my experiences I can help others, then it would be selfish to keep the story of how I beat my own alcoholism to myself, and so I will recount the awful things that I did, the often vile and abusive person that I became and the pain and worry that I put my loved ones through.

Even after I had cruelly hurt them and then begged for forgiveness – again, and they had forgiven me – again, and I promised that I would stop drinking – again, I would always, eventually drink that first alcoholic drink, (alcoholics say they 'pick up' again), and I would begin the journey back down the spiral.

In the earlier years, I would pick up a drink again b[illegible] would come to convince myself that this time it wou[illegible] different, this time I would be able to control it and drink i[illegible] 'normal' way. In the latter years, I kept on drinking even after[illegible] I had done something awful, because I just couldn't stop, because alcohol eventually became the only essential part of my life.

Sadly and predictably, every time I took that first drink after a period of abstinence, the descent down the spiral gathered pace and the damage that I caused to relationships and the hurt to those who loved me escalated.

While having to trawl back through my memories of the last 30 or so years, it struck me that, although it is clear that my alcoholism progressed through all of the well-documented stages, in the earlier years the timelines of those stages are blurred and each phase just gradually merges into the next. In fact, I'd even struggle to pin point which year it was that I deteriorated from being a problem drinker to becoming a functioning alcoholic, (early, middle and late stages).

In contrast, the escalation from being a functioning alcoholic to an alcoholic that just can't function and then becoming an end stage alcoholic whose time was running out, is much more obvious and happened alarmingly quickly, (late and end stages).

While the earlier timelines may be blurred, when I have now had to consider my drinking over the years for this book, what has become very clear to me is that my attitude to certain things makes them useful 'markers' of my descent down the spiral.

ıen reading through my timeline, that my
lrink driving and lying to those I love
y distorted. The list of things and events
with alcohol which made it 'legitimate' for
grew longer, the accidents that I had when
e more frequent and more serious, and the
rules I made for myself about what and when I could drink were constantly being re-written.

So, although the timelines are blurred, the way in which these 'markers' change over time, clearly illustrates the progression of my alcoholism, my moral decline and my descent into chaos.

I also now realise that I was drinking alcoholically for much longer than I ever admitted, because it's not how much you drink, but the motivation behind your drinking that differentiates an alcoholic from someone who simply likes a drink. Anyway, regardless of labels, I always drank too much and the fact that I frequently tried to curb my drinking, even years ago, indicates that deep down I knew I had a problem.

Although there are very few people about whom others would say, 'drinking alcohol really brings out the best in them', the loss of inhibition brought on by even a small amount of alcohol means that some people actually can benefit from having a drink to loosen them up and it can enable some people to relax in situations that they might otherwise be stressed about. Meeting new people or dancing at a party for example. A 'normal' person drinking alcohol will find that even a relatively small amount can relax them and this is one of the reasons why people have been drinking alcohol for thousands of years.

I always thought that I was one of those people, using alcohol to boost my confidence or to have a better time, but I can now see what those closest to me realised very quickly - nothing positive ever resulted from me drinking alcohol and I was kidding myself when I believed that it made me funnier, more articulate, more confident.... the list goes on. It was more likely to make me self-pitying, obnoxious, depressed, angry, reckless, cruel, embarrassing.... (not necessarily all at the same time!) and this got worse over the years. Even at a young age, I would often be that friend sitting in the corner crying and feeling sorry for myself after drinking too much - probably after doing something outrageous to make people laugh - as my friend Vicky put it years ago, 'you never know which Sue you're going to get'.

And that is how alcohol gets a grip. A person who starts out using it to be more confident or, (unknowingly), to mask parts of their personality or block out unpleasant feelings, finds that they need more and more alcohol over time to achieve the same effect, (their tolerance of alcohol goes up). But as we drink more alcohol, get drunk, binge drink, the changes to our personality and behaviour become increasingly negative and alcohol, which is actually a poison, becomes more and more toxic to us - physically, mentally and spiritually.

This brings me to an important point. I am, like a lot of alcoholics I have met, fundamentally a decent, caring person. Reading my timeline chronicling my descent into full blown alcoholism, you could be forgiven for believing that I am a completely selfish and uncaring person and an unfit mother and I know that I don't come out of this looking very good. But, as I have said earlier, this is not a vanity project and I have focused purely on my relationship with alcohol and what it did to my life. This isn't meant to be a life story because that would be boring.

There were many times when I wasn't drinking as much, (when it was 'dormant'), when I was fun and a very loving wife and mother, (before my drinking became a major problem, my husband Ross would joke that life with me was 'never boring'). Inside the majority of alcoholics there is still the person who existed before they discovered alcohol, who in my case was decent, caring and fun, which is why my family and friends kept giving me chances - they loved the real me, but hated the alcoholic me. Jekyll and Hyde is a perfect analogy, because the drink soaked, alcoholic me was a monster.

Finally, before I chronicle my alcoholic journey, it is so important for me personally to stress here that my son Michael and husband Ross, as well as my first husband Mark, like all families of alcoholics, went through their own various stages of trying to deal with my drinking and their own normality became distorted because of alcohol, especially in the later years.

In the world of an alcoholic, it tends to be only those people who are closest to them, partners and children, who are fully aware of how bad things have become, because it happens gradually and they try to keep it within the family, out of a sense of loyalty and also embarrassment. This is why the extent of the problem can come as a huge shock to even close friends and family outside of the actual home, who often only become aware when crisis point is reached.

The interventions of Ross and Michael and before them Mark, progressed from gentle and loving suggestions that I'd had enough to drink, to ultimately trying desperately to control my drinking through threats and arguments and throwing away alcohol that I had hidden.

They came to dread attending social events with me because my behaviour was always so unpredictable and then, in the end, Ross and Michael sadly and reluctantly adapted to living with me sleeping off a hangover, or being drunk and abusive during the day. They became completely defeated. 'Normality' in our household changed as my alcoholism took hold and I know that this made them feel deeply sad, totally powerless and very angry and frustrated, until ultimately my son was often placed in the tragic position where he felt that he had no option but to move out and live with his Dad Mark.

My son Michael has always been my world, which makes my alcoholism very difficult to understand and I still find it very difficult to think about what I put them all through.

Pre 1992

Before my mid 20's most people who knew me would probably say that, whilst I was a typical student who liked a blow out at weekends and sometimes suffered from horrible hangovers, drinking alcohol didn't really sit well with me. I would often end up crying or I would be full of angst and worry the next day about what I might have said or done.

Regardless of this, I certainly persevered with drinking and loved to drink to get drunk - I was never the sort of person who could just enjoy a couple of drinks and go home. I found very early on that alcohol made me feel more confident and I really enjoyed drinking.

Much to my embarrassment now, I won a drinking competition on the first night of my time at Durham University, by downing a pint of cider faster than the row of hopeful girls next to me, (I was living in an all-girls college at the university). The prize was to be crowned 'College Drunk' for the year which seemed hilarious at the time and simply good, innocent fun, but now it just seems quite sad and ominous.

The fact that I was one of the only people that I knew there to have come from a council house made me even more regretful about winning this title, because it made me a figure of fun and wasn't a true reflection of the immense pride that I felt having gained a place at such a prestigious university.

Even looking back to my Sixth Form Leavers Dinner, I was 'tipsy' when I gave my speech as Head Girl, because I had smuggled Cinzano into the school in a baby bottle and I drank it very quickly in the toilets with my friends.

I had never been one of those teenagers to hang around parks getting drunk, so this was actually very unusual for me, but I had never had to make a speech before either, and it made me feel very confident. After that I began to feel that drinking had the power to take away my inhibitions, making me confident and fun. All those years ago, I felt it improved me.

1992 - 1995

After graduating from Newcastle Business School, I got married to my childhood sweetheart Mark, (we actually got together at school in the sixth form) and we moved south with his job. I got a job in the Pharmaceutical Industry, which I found suited me really well because I loved promoting medicines to Doctors and I really liked the people that I worked with. However, like many industries in the 90's, there was a strong emphasis placed upon entertaining, which meant evening meetings as well as overnight stays.

At company conferences I would find myself surrounded by incredibly confident people, many of whom loved to drink. I happily joined in, mainly because I found that alcohol took away my nerves when I secretly, and mistakenly, felt out of my depth and intimidated due to my working class background. Alcohol definitely helped me to feel confident with my peers. I was popular and considered to be a good laugh, and joking about 'death by mini bar' after a heavy night became the norm.

Because I was relatively young, I found it easy to be one of the last people in the bar at night and then up early for meetings the next day, looking immaculate in my suit. It wasn't until I was pregnant with my son in 1995 and I gave up drinking, that I realised on a conference that I had to attend that there weren't actually that many very drunk people. I can remember saying to someone, 'where are all of the drunk reps, falling around and being a disgrace' and he laughed, 'it's usually only you, Sue!' which I also laughed off. At home though, when it was just me and Mark, I didn't drink during the week and we would share a bottle of wine on weekend evenings and we were very happy.

1995-1997

After the birth of our son Michael I went back to work pretty quickly. This was out of necessity rather than a desire to pursue a career - I absolutely adored my son and I loved being a Mum and I sobbed when I had to go back to work. However, I know that lots of women have to do this every day and so I just had to get on with it. My husband Mark worked very long hours and it was at this time that I found my best friend, who was not only a colleague but she had also given birth to a son six weeks before me. We became soul mates and I loved her, I still do, and we both adored our sons and both liked a glass of wine at each other's homes when our partners were working late and it was during this time that I began to sometimes drink 'on a school night'.

I would love to parcel Michael up on a Friday evening and take him over to her house to stay, knowing that I could drink wine at the same time as planning our future around our boys and talking about how we were so lucky to have them within weeks of each other and how they would grow up to be best friends....... We would dance around her kitchen and laugh harder than I have ever laughed and it seemed like such innocent fun, with the boys cheerfully playing together and dancing with us - but I sometimes drank too much and deep down I knew that I was being irresponsible.

However, I always congratulated myself that I could never quite finish a second bottle of wine and this was my unspoken rule and reassurance, meaning that I couldn't possibly have a drink problem.

Anyway, I was also working full time and in my mind alcoholics didn't have jobs and, because I had a high pressured sales job, I was entitled to let my hair down and relax. It didn't cross my mind that I was choosing to spend my free time doing this, rather than being with Mark, but I can see now that this is because Mark didn't like the effect that alcohol had on my personality and liked us to do other things- but I loved how alcohol made me feel. Without me realising it, I was already making unconscious decisions, and very important ones at that, based around alcohol and my love of 'escape' and in my mind I wasn't doing any harm – I was just a working mum, relaxing and letting off steam.

But there were some afternoons, when I would meet colleagues after work before I went home, at some pretty little bistro, (even then I believed that alcoholics don't go to nice bistros!), when I would definitely be over the limit to drive and I always made a promise to myself never to let this happen again. At the same time as I was discovering my love of a nice Sancerre, (again, I believed that posh wine isn't the drink of alcoholics), my husband Mark was becoming increasingly concerned about my drinking and it would cause arguments. I wasn't drinking every day, but it was the effect that alcohol had on my personality that upset him.

I saw his attempts at suggesting that I drank too much or that it changed my 'lovely' personality as him trying to control me and I used that to turn myself against him. He loved the real Susan and I can remember him clearly trying to explain to me that when we were out he would just 'lose' the real me half way through the evening and he hated it. I increasingly became the angry or self-pitying version of myself, who wanted to drink because 'I felt guilty about leaving my son in a nursery all day and that was his fault', or one of the many other excuses I would use for having a bottle of wine.

In fact, I now see that I would create a drama, engineer a crisis or go on a guilt trip as an excuse to drink and that alcohol, even then, was beginning to turn me into a master manipulator. I still feel a deep sense of shame because Michael was an absolute breeze as a baby and I know that Mark loved me very much but what I didn't realise, or didn't want to acknowledge, was that alcohol was beginning to become more and more important in my life even then.

1997-2001

After having a brief separation from Mark, (following an alcohol fuelled argument), we got back together and I moved to a new company for a fresh start. I had admitted to Mark that there had been times that I was worried about my drinking and I did try to make rules about when I could drink and I would try to do things like alternating between wine and soft drinks when we were out. I loved him and loved my son more than anything and I knew that my behaviour when I had a drink was upsetting for them both. Eventually, after a couple of glasses of wine, I would make jokes that I was alternating red wine with white wine and my rules would go out of the window - but it wasn't funny and it humiliated Mark on many occasions.

Once I had had a couple of glasses of wine I felt so different – I felt confident, funny, daring, outgoing and attractive and I never had an 'off' switch. In between my fun drinking times I became more and more bitter and angry about my life as a working Mum, but I only understood years later that alcohol is a depressant and it was my excessive drinking that was making me feel low, not the fact that my son was in nursery while I worked - that was just an excuse that I could use to justify having a drink and punish my husband for.

During these years I had a bad fall down some stairs while I was drunk and was told in the hospital while they were stitching my chin, (I had landed on my chin and it had taken the full force of the fall), that it was a miracle that I hadn't broken my neck. Mark and I also had a romantic break in Paris one time and I drunkenly climbed out of the window of our fourth floor hotel room, thinking it was funny to scare him by sitting on the window ledge. All through that time, I never thought I had a drink problem and I never saw that alcohol was damaging my life and I became increasingly defensive about it.

There were so many occasions during this time where I spoiled a special event (including Michael's Christening), embarrassed myself and Mark or did and said cruel and hurtful things (always when I was drunk) and Mark always forgave me. He called it my 'Jekyll and Hyde', because when I wasn't drinking, I was a totally different person.

Mark then had an opportunity to move back up north to run his family's company and he was excited to make a fresh start for our little family. It was then that I made a devastating and unforgivable decision and told him that I would not be moving with him because I had established my own career, but I see now that this was partly because subconsciously a life without him there to control my drinking and 'fun' seemed more appealing. The fact that I was breaking his heart and breaking up our family didn't sway me, because I, (and alcohol), had convinced myself that our marriage wasn't working.

This was definitely when alcohol, very quietly, started to run my life, but it would take me years to realise this.

During this time I changed jobs again and bought a house for me and my son. My niece moved down from the North East to live in with us and help with the school run, so that I could work. I was proud of the fact that I was a strong, independent woman who could survive as a single parent and I loved having friends over to stay sometimes and my drinking generally cranked up a notch. I would frequently be hungover and most likely over the limit driving to work, but I would love the fact that I could have a bottle of wine every night with no one to stop me and I know that this was not easy for my niece.

My son was about five by then and I remember becoming aware that he didn't like it when he saw me with a drink, and I would sometimes hide my wine bottles from Michael or drink wine out of a mug, so that my little boy could not tell that I was drinking. The fact that I saw this as a practical solution and nothing out of the ordinary is now unbelievable to me, but it made perfect sense at the time. I remember vividly one day when I had a glass of wine in my hand and Michael said to me, 'Mummy, I like it when you drink tea', because even at that young age, he knew that my personality changed when I was drinking wine.

After one very alarming, unforgivable and sobering event when I had been hungover and deeply asleep in bed and Michael had let himself out of the house one morning, I decided to try to cut down, (not give up completely), and I went to see my GP because, for that brief moment in time, I was concerned that I might have a problem. I was referred to a counsellor and went for a few sessions, but I quickly came to the conclusion that I wasn't actually as bad as I had thought and that I had overreacted, (this was to become a cycle of behaviour), and that I would be able to control my drinking all by myself.

So began many attempts at trying to curb my drinking, usually after I did something that frightened me, but I never felt that things were bad enough for me to give up alcohol altogether.

2001 - 2005

It became increasingly obvious to me that I had been very pig headed and stupid to stay in the south with Michael, when Mark and my own large family lived in the north. I realised that I needed a support network and so I sold my house and prepared for the move. At a pharmaceutical meeting one night before I moved, I bumped into Ross, (who is now my husband), and we hit it off straight away. I explained that I was moving up north and had sold my house and that I couldn't start a serious relationship and I went ahead and made the move in time for Michael to start the new school year. Ross began to travel up north to see us, our relationship developed and I started another job in Newcastle - I felt that life was good and I was making a fresh start.

I was still drinking alone most nights, but because this had been gradual and had now gone on for so long, and because I was holding down a job, I didn't regard it as a problem – it relaxed me and made me switch off.

Ross eventually decided to move north to be with us and my relationship with Mark, who was now in a serious relationship himself and very happy, was friendly and supportive because of Michael.

However, very gradually, my alcohol consumption began to creep up. The fact that I could never physically drink two bottles of wine in one session in the past had always made me believe that I didn't have an alcohol problem, but over time I began to realise that some nights I was easily drinking two bottles. It wasn't every night, but there had definitely been a change in my tolerance levels – although not enough for me to avoid hangovers.

At about the same time I quit the job I was doing in Newcastle because I hated not being able to do the school run and to meet Michael at the school gates every afternoon, and I felt that this was more important than having a well-paid job. I wanted to be there for Michael and to be a proper Mum and Ross was very supportive, but this also made it easy for me to not have to worry about a fuzzy head the next day and, although it wasn't a deliberate move on my part to be able to drink more, in retrospect it certainly made it easier.

Around this time I also occasionally felt the need to have a miniature bottle of wine before an event for 'Dutch Courage', like meeting Mark at Michael's school play, which I'd never done before. Again, I normalised this and brushed it off as calming my nerves or allowing me to appear confident, because I found the mothers at Michael's school intimidating and I wanted to appear just as confident and glamorous as them. In retrospect it's surprising how this soon became the norm for me when preparing for many events, or just meeting people in general.

Over these years we had many great parties at our house and I loved being a hostess and giving people a fun time, but I would always drink far too much and end up worrying the next day about what I might have said or done. I never, ever had an 'off' switch with alcohol and I would be envious of people like Ross who could enjoy a drink and even, on occasion, get drunk, but could switch to water before getting completely out of control.

I would always convince myself that I could be like this too, but on most occasions, once I'd had a few drinks, I would drink until I had to be put to bed.

I simply never, ever learned and I loved the feeling that drinking gave me – I wanted to stay up and dance all night but I'd more often than not end up in an emotional heap. I also cracked ribs and split my head several times with drunken falls, but told myself that everyone has accidents like that at some point.

The morning after, I would often be embarrassed or worried because I couldn't remember events from the night before. It's as if the saying 'drinking today steals happiness from tomorrow' was created for me.

Then something changed. I went from being comfortable with my 'liking a drink' and 'maybe drinking too much' and seeing myself as a fun, party person, to feeling a bit uneasy about how much I was actually drinking. The nightly bottle of wine changed to a nightly bottle and a half of wine and increasingly regular 'blow outs' with two or three bottles of wine.

But, probably the most alarming development was my first experimentation with 'hair of the dog'. I had never needed or wanted alcohol in the morning before, but on this particular day in the midst of an awful hangover, I remembered that I had promised to drive my sister Eileen to the Metrocentre, a large shopping centre in town. I decided that a gulp of wine would shift my hangover and I took a really good swig before I set off to pick her up, with Michael in the car with me.

She was absolutely furious. She suspected immediately that I had been drinking and she tackled me about it as soon as we got to the Metrocentre, only after she had had to brave a journey with me driving and risking her life and the lives of our kids. I was mortified, sorry and ashamed and couldn't believe that I had been so irresponsible and reckless, and I promised her and everyone else that I would get help. I searched for a hypnotherapist on the internet and went to see someone who assured me that they could definitely stop me from drinking alcohol - and I did stop for a while.

But it didn't last for long and things were only going to get much worse.

Chapter 2

Problem Drinking To Functioning Alcoholic

After the 'hair of the dog' incident, when I recklessly chose to drive with my sister and our kids in the car, alcohol very gradually took over my life completely. Over the next eight years, I became firmly shackled onto the tracks of the hellish descent that alcohol takes some people down, only it was a slow ride.

Sometimes, usually after seeing a hypnotherapist, counsellor or trying AA for a while, I managed to convince myself - and others - that I had jumped off, pulled myself together and could even drink 'normally' again.

And that is one of the many cruel and deceptive things about alcohol - an alcoholic can have months and even years of sobriety or even 'normal' drinking, but the dark shadow of alcoholism is always there hiding in the background, waiting to make a move.

Also, no matter how low alcohol takes a person and how many promises they make about never drinking again, as well as knowing how much they will lose if they ever do drink again, alcohol cunningly convinces the alcoholic that this time it will be different, this time they will somehow regain control. The dark shadow whispers to them and lies to them. And then the hideous, boring and destructive cycle begins again.

Over the following eight years I slowly began to be secretive about my drinking. My family and friends were occasionally concerned about how drunk I got at parties or other social gatherings and they 'never knew what they were going to get', but I would try to distract everyone from focusing on my drinking by creating dramas or by exaggerating issues in my life. I also became increasingly defensive if anyone mentioned how much I drank, so that they eventually became scared to say anything. For a long time those around me had no idea that I often indulged in 'hidden drinking' before an event, or even at an event, where I was also socially drinking with everyone.

I know that many people can innocently enjoy a glass of wine or their favourite alcoholic drink while they are getting ready for an event and that this is often part of the fun and the ritual of preparing to go out, but I began to believe that I couldn't meet people socially or attend an event without having had a drink or, increasingly, a few drinks beforehand to loosen me up. This meant that it often appeared that I simply couldn't drink as much as other people, because I would get drunk relatively quickly compared to them, when all along the reality was that I had probably had more than double or treble the amount of wine my friends and family thought I'd had.

Although this started as my way of 'getting in the mood' or conquering my imaginary nerves, it gradually crept into my life until it became completely normal for me to drink a bottle or more of wine while I put my makeup on for a night out. It is incredible how alcoholics can always justify their own drinking to themselves and I would always convince myself that I was doing no harm, because other people indulged in 'pre drinks', and they would laugh about it on social media.

I also told myself that the people around me didn't know the full extent of the pressures I was under and what I was dealing with in my life, (nothing more than anyone else as it happens), which justified my drinking to me. I even believed that, because no one would understand or believe that I was completely in control of my drinking, it was better for them that they did not know the true amount of alcohol that I was consuming, because it would only worry them since they would be judging me relative to their own tolerance levels etc. I honestly felt that what they didn't know couldn't harm them and that I was actually protecting them from unnecessary worry.

For a long time I managed to maintain some semblance of normality for Michael and Ross and would pride myself on always cooking a family dinner every night, (always with a glass of wine at hand, which seemed sophisticated and homely and, in my head, was what other women did, - but then eventually with bottle of wine hidden somewhere else).

I also invented and brought to market a product in the middle of this period, (as my counsellor in one rehab said, 'god knows what you could've done with that business if you'd been sober'), which I believed was proof that I couldn't possibly have a drink problem.

However, over time my life between 2005 and 2013 became increasingly chaotic. I seemed to be frequently facing a drama or a crisis, which I can now see were manufactured as smokescreens to divert attention from my drinking, as well as providing me with valid excuses to drink because I was 'upset'. I also began to hide more and more alcohol from everyone.

Eventually, where I used to love going to social events, I came to dread them, because I felt everyone would be clocking what I was drinking, and so I began to pretend I wasn't drinking at all, to 'prove' that I didn't have a problem. Sadly on those occasions, I would invariably have a secret stash of alcohol in my handbag to drink in the toilet or outside.

In later years I would avoid social events altogether and began to isolate myself, because I knew that I would almost certainly make a complete fool of myself and embarrass everyone and, because I didn't want to risk doing that, I preferred to stay in and drink at home. Towards the end of this period, I simply stopped being able to trust myself to go out and have a good time, because I accepted that I had zero control over alcohol.

I don't know why or how alcohol went from being something that gave me confidence to being something I began to be embarrassed about and to hide from people, but I do know that I always felt a massive sense of relief when I was drinking and reassured when I knew I had a supply of alcohol available to me. I loved the fact that drinking took away my cares and worries.

The fact that many of my worries over the years were a direct result of my drinking never really registered with me. Alcohol became a friend to me and it got to the point where I would associate everything with alcohol to justify having a drink. Happy times, sad times, celebrations, sunny days, cold winter nights - everything painted a picture in my head of a lovely scene with the appropriate alcoholic drink in hand.

Because there were periods of time over these years when I managed to get a grip on my drinking, there were many happy times for Ross, Michael and me, we even had fun parties where I could be on top form, the proverbial life and soul.

We also had some lovely family holidays together over these years, but my drinking and the feelings behind it increasingly interrupted our lives and began to really scare me. I came to live in fear of being found out and of forgetting what I might have said or done when I'd had a drink, because I frequently had complete 'blanks' about the night before, (known as a 'black out').

This became a familiar pattern when I would have to subtly 'check in' with people the day after an evening of drinking, to gauge whether I had upset them and I would be frantic with panic and incredibly anxious if I couldn't get in contact with people.

Each time I woke up after having upset someone or embarrassed myself by throwing up, falling down in public or being nasty, once I had 'checked in' with people to apologise and to reassure myself that I had got away with it and was in the clear so to speak, I would have exactly the same conversation with myself. This would be along the lines of, 'okay, you got away with it this time. That was the last time. Pull yourself together now and act normally, then everyone will forget and think it was a one off……'

I can imagine my dark shadow attempting to high five me to congratulate me on getting away with it, but I always just felt wretched and embarrassed and in no mood to look upon these events as any kind of victory.

As these years passed, I increasingly cancelled events and meetings and let people down, either because I was hungover or had been too drunk to prepare properly for a meeting or for seeing friends.

Again, this turned into a pattern and gradually became my 'normal', with more and more elaborate lies and excuses - a sordid and secretive life. I became completely selfish, self-pitying and self-absorbed and ruled by alcohol, but what I desperately wanted to do was to get back to how I used to be, when drinking was fun and I was happy. For this reason I could not consider giving up alcohol completely and would constantly try to control my drinking and make new 'rules' for myself, (when I could drink, where I could drink, alternating days on and off alcohol etc.), but my rules were quickly broken and frequently re written.

I blamed my unhappiness on everyone and everything and looked for answers and reasons - even convincing myself that I was going through an early menopause which must have caused a hormonal imbalance, ultimately resulting in my excessive drinking, and I insisted on a referral from my GP to see a gynaecologist, when all I really needed was simple sobriety.

Alcohol does operate with stealth and has 'time and patience' and the changes in my drinking and behaviour were so gradual over these years, that they became normal. I also had periods of time when I didn't drink, usually after a drunken event had frightened me and those around me. Between 2005 and 2013, I paid to see five different hypnotherapists, had counselling and went to AA meetings, (I talk about these in later chapters), only to convince myself time and time again that these were knee-jerk reactions to a 'mishap' that could have happened to anyone.

Most importantly, over this time I completely lost any sense of who I really was and how much love I had around me.

Autumn 2005

The day before Michael's tenth birthday, I had a particularly hideous hangover and somehow convinced myself once more that 'hair of the dog' would sort me out and make me feel human again. Michael had been staying with Mark and, unusually for me, I had been drinking vodka the night before with friends who didn't know I was developing a serious problem. The next morning I thought that I could cure my hangover with a gulp of vodka, but I was mainly used to drinking wine and I drank the vodka in the same greedy way, gulping it down in the same quantity. I quickly passed out, completely drunk.

When I eventually came around, hours had passed, the whole day had gone and it was almost school pick up time. I knew there was no way that I was fit to drive anywhere and so I rang Michael's auntie and asked her to pick him up, also asking if he could stay with her that night as a treat. I told myself that I could pick him up from school the next day, his birthday, and everything would be fine and no one would be any the wiser. However she knew immediately that there must be something very wrong, because the real me would never have dreamed of missing out on waking up with Michael on his tenth birthday.

Ross was away, so she rang Mark, who then rang my sister Eileen, and they both came to the house to see what the problem was. Unfortunately, before they arrived I had decided to drink even more vodka because I felt so sorry for myself and ashamed at missing Michael's birthday morning, which resulted in me passing out in an alcohol induced 'coma'. Because I was unconscious, I didn't hear them frantically ringing the doorbell, calling me on my phone and hammering on the windows – they were desperately worried.

They finally managed to break into the house and thought that I was dead when they first found me in bed. I was completely out of it when I woke up and began crying and pleading with them not to think badly of me, but I was still completely intoxicated. Eileen ended up having to stay the night and the next day she and our sister Patricia took me to see my GP, with a list worries about my drinking. I was hungover and ashamed, and begged him to prescribe me Antabuse, a medication for alcoholics, which I was convinced would stop me from drinking because of the violent physical reaction that you experience if you drink alcohol whilst you are taking it.

I realised then that I definitely needed help and that my drinking was out of control, and I booked myself into my first rehab, which I only went to for two weeks, (more of this in Chapter 5). However, when I left rehab I managed to convince myself and Ross that I was 'cured'. I decided I had nothing remotely resembling the problems of the other people I had met whilst I was there, but I had learned a valuable lesson, and I told myself that my new perspective would allow me to drink socially again and I could put the past behind me.

2006 - 2007

I really was determined that I was going to draw a line under everything and start afresh - and I did, for a while. I honestly felt that the 'vodka incident' and rehab afterwards had been a big mistake, that we had all over reacted and I tried very hard to be a 'normal' drinker, (although my normal drinking was still at least one bottle of wine per night, sometimes more).

I got a job in a café near our house, and took Michael to join a local football team. I threw myself into the role of being a football Mum, only to discover, (to my delight), that the other parents of the team loved to drink and party. The football soon became a sideshow for me while we all enjoyed socialising together and looking back I am ashamed when I remember the football tournaments where the efforts and achievements of the boys playing football became secondary to our socialising, and I often found myself drinking until I was blind drunk.

After several incidents which ranged from embarrassing to unforgivable, I again decided that I had a problem with alcohol that I needed to sort out. The mild things were worrying enough, such as frequently waking up after a football tournament, awards ceremony or 'team bonding' football social in total blackout, with no memory of the evening before and in a massive panic.

Then there was the time I fell asleep in the airport toilets after a football trip before our flight, drunk from the night before and also the occasional secret sips of cooking brandy that I drank in the store cupboard of the café where I worked to help cure a hangover, or to get me through a boring day.

I also delighted in starting conversations with complete strangers when I was out with Ross, convinced that they would be so interested in what I had to say, when they just wanted to be left alone to get on with their own evening. I was embarrassing and boring and Ross hated it and dreaded going anywhere with me if it meant I would be drinking.

Other incidents were far more serious, including drunkenly starting a fight with a woman at Ross' company Christmas party because I thought that she fancied him, (after which I begged Ross for forgiveness and promised I wouldn't drink again). The whole thing was excruciatingly embarrassing for Ross, not to mention potentially career limiting, but after lots of champagne and wine I felt that I needed to confront her and she needed to have the (imaginary) smug smile wiped off her face. It didn't cross my mind how this would impact on Ross, (who had to write a formal apology, but it could have been much worse).

I increasingly risked driving my car when I knew that I was over the limit and on one occasion I drove to my Mum's house worse for wear which really frightened her. And so, because I became concerned about my drinking again and terrified of losing Ross and Michael, I arranged a session with another hypnotherapist who promised to turn me off alcohol completely, which I so desperately wanted. It failed.

Despite the Christmas Party incident, Ross and I got married in the summer of 2006. I found that I managed to control my drinking around the time of the wedding and our honeymoon, and the months before and after were a very happy time for the three of us.

Michael escorted me into the chapel and I was so proud of him, my best friend did a reading and I felt very lucky to have found, (and kept), Ross. I became confident again that I didn't have an alcohol problem, as alcoholics do, because I had managed not to get drunk on our wedding day, and my 'controlled' drinking continued until 2007. I still drank too much and would hide the amount that I drank, but I believed that I had it under control and that I could live this way forever.

Then, almost one year after our wedding, my darling best friend died very suddenly. I was completely devastated, and it sent me into overwhelming shock and grief that I hadn't ever experienced before. I loved her, she was a truly special person, and we had recently spoken about growing older as best friends, visiting each other for Christmases and spending long summer weekends together with our boys. I was genuinely bereft when she died, but after her death I would wallow in self-pity, crying into my wine, convincing myself that this was 'normal' behaviour, and I knew that I would never be challenged by Ross, because he was sensitive to the fact that I was grieving for my friend.

But weeks of this became months and I found myself hiding bottles again and drinking more than my 'official' daily allowance of wine, and I would frequently need to ask Ross to do the school run because I was too hungover. This is still very difficult for me to come to terms with, even now, because the school run, when I had Michael all to myself in the car twice a day, was my absolutely favourite time. I loved talking to him and listening to his music and the fact that I would choose to sacrifice that for a drink is tragic, and makes me feel incredibly ashamed and heavyhearted because I can never have those times back.

Ross and my close friends eventually voiced their concerns about my behaviour, (on more than one occasion I turned up to meet my friends for lunch drunk after driving there, and every time I met them I would order Long Island Iced Tea, because I understood that it was the most alcoholic cocktail) and I agreed, again, that I needed to seek help and began to go to AA meetings. My friend Paula came with me to the first meeting for moral support and I felt a real sense of relief that I was doing something about my drinking.

2008

Predictably, after going to AA for a while, I decided again that I was not an alcoholic because the people that I met there had far worse problems than I did, and I believed I would never be like them. I am ashamed that I also convinced Ross, again, that I could control my drinking and that I had just been drinking more, temporarily, because I was grieving for my friend. Because Ross loves me so much, he wanted to believe me and so I began another cycle of trying to drink normally, sometimes hiding drinks, having long periods of time of relative normality, with occasional completely insane episodes, (climbing onto our conservatory crying in the middle of the night; threatening to say I had a bomb on an aircraft at the beginning of what was meant to be a lovely holiday to Egypt for the three of us, being verbally abusive to strangers).

I look back on these events and I cringe because alcohol had the most profound effect on my personality – it basically turned me into a crazy woman – but I never thought that then, the things I did made perfect sense or seemed funny at that moment in time.

I always had an excuse or would try to laugh things off, and even though my behaviour under the influence was by then often dangerous and always completely embarrassing, I still felt that drinking improved me in some way, or made me feel happier and more fun. My friends and family were also giving me another chance and I was able to drink socially in front of them again, but I remember staying at my friend Vicky's and hiding vodka in my bag because she drinks very little, and I anticipated that she probably wouldn't be pouring the wine fast enough for me.

I was losing all sense of right and wrong and respect for people, and I was losing myself. I didn't understand what was happening to me.

In the summer of 2008 our home was flooded and we had to move out for six months - something that happens to many people and they just get on with it, (as Ross and Michael had to do). Unsurprisingly this was my cue to wallow in self-pity and ramp up my drinking again – drunkenly persuading Michael to help me smash up a 'Nefertiti' bust that we had bought on holiday, because I was (drunkenly) convinced it was cursed and had caused the flood.

We chose to rent a house closer to Michael's school for the six months that it took to repair the flood damage, (we lived in the country and Michael's school was in the city). We saw this as a treat for Michael, and felt it would soften the blow for him that our house was in such a mess, because it meant that he could walk to and from the school with his friends. Inadvertently, this also meant that I didn't have to worry about the guilt of not doing the school run anymore and so hangovers didn't matter. My drinking again stepped up a notch and I found myself drinking earlier in the day.

I had given up my job in the café and I would find myself shopping and then having wine in Marks and Spencer's café, telling myself that wine with lunch was acceptable and did not mean I was an alcoholic. I then discovered their handy little cans of cocktails, which I began to buy because they were easy to hide in my bag. I cannot explain why this started to happen, but at the time I know that it seemed to make perfect sense, and I began to love my new life living in the city and having a 'cocktail' during the day – the fact that I might drink that cocktail in the toilets of Marks and Spencer because I couldn't wait until I got home didn't seem alarming.

Predictably, this new found daytime drinking started to impact on my life at home. I was frequently lying to Ross about what I'd done during the day, and I noticed that Michael was spending more time with his friends and would often look dejected – but alcoholic me put this down to the fact that he was now a moody teenager. However, after yet another drunken episode when I became vile and belligerent with Mark on the phone and Michael was upset with me, I promised Michael and Ross, again, that I would seek help. I went to see my GP, who sent me for counselling and acupuncture.

This lasted for a few months and life again became more stable and happy for a while, and I felt that I was in control again. When I met my counsellor I would wear a suit, so that I looked respectable and, in my mind, the opposite of how one might suppose an alcoholic would look (I can now imagine my dark shadow helping me choose what to wear to fool her). I would say what she wanted to hear and lie that I had given up drink completely, and eventually I decided that I didn't need to see her anymore.

2009 - 2010

When we moved back into our house I threw myself into developing my invention, an idea I had had for a while, and which I had convinced Ross would be our ticket to wealth and happiness. This involved re-mortgaging our house for the initial investment and taking huge financial risks, but I thought that it would create happiness for us because I was sure that I would be so busy working on it that I wouldn't have time to be a problem drinker again, and I certainly wouldn't have time for days lost to hangovers.

I was determined to make it a success and to make Ross and Michael proud of me again - and even get some self-respect back. What I should have realised was that all that they truly wanted was normality and calm and predictability - and for me to stop drinking completely.

My grand gesture of inventing something and being a businesswoman was not even slightly important or impressive to them - they just wanted the real me back and some stability in their lives.

By now I had convinced everyone, (or so I thought), that I was not a 'proper' alcoholic by explaining that I had occasionally used alcohol as a crutch in the past, to get me through tough times, and that lots of other people do this from time to time too.

I was even happy to blame my behaviour on mental health issues, which is something that some alcoholics do, because we would rather blame our behaviour on anything other than having a problem with alcohol.

I got to know some local women through walking our dog Mutley and we began to walk our dogs together, becoming close friends. Our walks were something that I really enjoyed and looked forward to but, as with other things in my life, I became increasingly unreliable because of my drinking and hangovers, and I would tell lies to them about missing walks because I was so ashamed.

I tried very hard to stay sober when we met people socially, but I had so many days at home where I would have an awful hangover because I had again drank secretly the night before on top of the 'official' wine that I could have in front of Ross. Because of this, I began to use 'hair of the dog' more and more to get to meetings, and I was frequently drunk when I met people and often over the limit when I was driving.

I know now that the people I was dealing with in business meetings would have realised this, or that they probably, at best, thought that I was quite highly strung, but I believed then that I was very good at hiding the fact that I had been drinking. I once threw up over myself in the car in a carpark before a meeting, which I had to cancel and go home, but somehow I convinced myself that this was an unfortunate 'one off' and not a major cause for concern.

Michael was a teenager by now and had got used to me being unpredictable when he got home from school, and he got on with his own life with his sports and his friends. I am ashamed to admit that he once reluctantly mentioned to me that his bedding wasn't clean and his friends joked about the spiders webs in his bedroom, because housework frequently became too much of an effort for me.

I used to convince him and Ross that I needed a drink on an evening to get through the stresses of getting my product to market. I couldn't possibly have a drink problem because I was a businesswoman who went to meetings with intelligent, important people and looked smart in her suit. If they ever suspected that I had had a drink, I would convince them that I had taken water retention tablets which had made me light headed, or I was pre-menstrual or peri-menopausal - in fact anything alluding to sensitive 'women's problems', which I knew they wouldn't challenge me over and didn't want to hear about.

Even when I was trying to convince them again that I wasn't drinking excessively, I knew that I had my secret stash of wine bottles hidden around the house and probably some cans of cocktails or gin and tonics in my handbag. In fact, without me realising it, those hidden bottles and cans had become a necessity now, and it gave me a calming reassurance to know that there was always a drink available if I needed one.

I even bought a breathalyser on the internet to demonstrate to them that I was happy to be breathalysed at any time, but they never used it because by then they were getting to the stage where they were mentally switching off to me, and ceasing to care or believe anything that I said. I also spent a fortune on vitamins in a vain attempt to try to cancel out the harmful effects of alcohol and to protect my liver and overall health.

I believed that I could go on like this forever and that I would never become one of those people whose drinking would escalate or be out of control.

There were some occasions during this time when Ross would have to make excuses to friends about why we couldn't meet them, because I had got myself into a state, and that is how it is for the families of alcoholics - they find themselves protecting the alcoholic out of loyalty and shame.

Ross especially covered for me with my family and friends and even Michael, more times than I know. He showed me nothing but love and I repaid him by attacking him verbally when I was drunk and blaming him for the 'stress' that made me drink. Deep down he was worried sick but also very angry. I constantly accused him of being unfaithful when he was away with work, and was jealous and insecure about his female colleagues. His life with me became intolerable, but all the while he had to continue to present the image of a focused professional in his pressured and highly responsible job.

On the occasions where we did see people, I would usually be embarrassing and I once fell into the millrace, (a very deep channel of water at the side of our garden), when we had people over for dinner. I had taken the dog out and everyone was inside our house and I could easily have drowned because I was so drunk. I walked back into the house soaking wet and covered in mud and leaves and went to bed without a word, leaving Ross alone with our guests.

We would visit people and I would find myself vomiting in secret throughout the evening, because any alcohol I had merely topped up my excesses from the night before and made me feel severely ill.

I also lost one of my oldest friends forever during this time when she turned up at my house as a lovely surprise, (she lived at the other end of the country). Ross was away with work and I was at home drunk. I told her that she had ruined my life because of an incident at school years before - I have never seen or heard from her since, even though I tried many times, which is tragic for me but completely understandable.

In fact my head was gradually filled with a proliferation of vile thoughts, paranoia and conspiracy theories when I was drunk. My dark shadow whispered venomous bile into my ear about people not liking me or laughing at me behind my back, or women flirting with Ross, or even just that I was a massive failure and worthless. This steadily got worse, but I didn't connect my negativity to alcohol and I was often very down because I felt so bad about everything.

Panic about my drinking would set in from time to time and this gradually developed into a constant, horrible gnawing feeling that just wouldn't go away - I started to feel really scared, but most of all I started to absolutely hate myself and I felt really ugly inside. I felt like nothing was real anymore, because I had this big secret and was living a complete lie, but I was frightened to tell anyone the truth.

I wanted so much to go back to a time when I could share a bottle of wine on a Saturday night and no more. Once again I arranged to see another hypnotherapist, this time over one hundred miles away and I visited them for at least four sessions, until I eventually felt that I was in control again.

2011- Early 2013

Somehow, and I don't know how, I launched my business in the spring of 2011, but my jubilation was cut short when my Dad very sadly and suddenly died the following day. Again, predictably, this became an excuse to increase my drinking to 'numb the pain' and I would sit up into the early hours listening to sad songs because in my mind 'that is what grieving people do'.

Yet again, Ross and Michael were put in a position where they didn't want to challenge my behaviour because my Dad had just died, but by then they were sick of my behaviour, and I started to hide alcohol even more. In a heart-breaking act of love and desperation, Michael bought me the book The Secret, which explains that everything you have ever wanted to be or achieve is within you, and I cried when I realised what I was doing to him and Ross.

Michael had by now passed his driving test, so I didn't need to do the school run any more. I also mourned this and the end of our regular journeys together, as a drama queen alcoholic does, even though there had been all of those times in the past when I had asked Ross to take him to school because I was too hungover or over the limit to drive.

I stumbled through the year dealing with the business and turning up to meetings over the limit. My life became increasingly out of control and I know that if it hadn't been for the fact that I was working for myself, I would definitely have been sacked.

If Ross and I stayed anywhere, the alcohol in the miniatures in the minibar would eventually be replaced by water, so he wouldn't know I'd been secretly drinking them, and I would often ruin a lovely time for him. I desperately wanted Ross and Michael to think that I wasn't drinking, and I desperately tried to make rules to stay sober - but I would still never consider giving it up completely.

I thought that alcohol gave me confidence and made me fun, (even then!), and I was still sure that I could get back to drinking normally again.

Because I hadn't enjoyed my experiences at AA meetings and I considered counselling to be a complete waste of time for me, I saw two more hypnotherapists over this time, (more of this in Chapter 4). They both guaranteed results but were both a total waste of money, as was my spending on vitamins and supplements in a vain attempt to protect myself against the physical harm that excessive drinking does.

After my business had been up and running for a while, I managed to secure a major investment, (Ross did all of the preparation work for the meeting), which meant that I could employ my sister Jane to help me with the day to day running of the business, while I spent my time trying to get retailers on board and generally promoting it.

It's amazing how many people come out of the woodwork when you have money to spend, and I found myself being talked into making bad business decisions and agreeing to spend money on things that, in retrospect, were unnecessary and frivolous - but I only have myself to blame because my head was often fuzzy and the alcohol clouded my judgement.

I loved working with Jane and being an 'entrepreneur' and feeling important, like I was actually achieving something, but I always believed that the people I met in relation to the business were my friends and had my best interests at heart. I was never thick skinned or discerning enough to be truly successful. How quickly they all melted away when the money ran out.

But for a few months during this time, I was also really happy. I absolutely loved working with my sister, we had such great times and some exciting triumphs with our little company. She was always supportive and I know that she covered for me on many occasions when I had a bad hangover or had a drink at a 'lunch meeting'. I joined an entrepreneurs group and generally tried to straighten myself out by becoming involved with a local charity. I really felt that I was close to getting my drinking more under control and making a success of myself.

I still drank secretly sometimes and always before I met 'important people' for my own confidence, but I believed that I was over the worst and would eventually be completely normal, especially when my business really took off, which I believed it eventually would. I was invited to give talks by the entrepreneurs group and asked to become an 'Angel of The North' on local radio, (their equivalent of Loose Women) and I genuinely believed that I could never have achieved any of this if I was an alcoholic.

Sadly, it was not to last. The investment company eventually said that my business could no longer afford staff, so I had the heart-breaking discussion with Jane. I was devastated for us both. It was one of the most difficult things I have ever had to do in my life, and it hit me and my sister incredibly hard.

Admittedly, this was a massive disappointment and a very tough time, but turning to alcohol robbed me of any perspective and it felt like the end of the world to me.

Wallowing in self-pity, my feelings of being a worthless failure were all-consuming; my dark shadow wrapped around me, and then that was it. This really was the beginning of the end for me, when alcohol made its devastating move, took over my life completely like a parasite, and went in for the kill.

Chapter 3

Functioning Alcoholic to an Alcoholic Who Couldn't Function

The following twenty or so months can only be described as a living nightmare and this has probably been the most difficult part of the book for me to write, because it was during this time that I went past the point of no return. Even though things actually got worse after this period, (Chapter 7 - Rock Bottom), between early 2013 and summer 2014 I crossed over an invisible line after which alcohol completely took control of my life, eventually becoming the most important thing to me, resulting in the most damaging and dangerous behaviour of my drinking existence.

I became a shell of a person, unable to enjoy anything because of the obsession that preoccupied my thoughts and the deep guilt and shame that never went away and the dark shadow consumed me completely.

Although I had been on my journey down the alcoholic spiral for years, things suddenly escalated at an alarming rate. Alcohol and being drunk became such an obsession that I eventually began to drink vodka like I used to drink wine, in gulps out of a bottle.

I can't blame this on the fact that my business wasn't doing well, because my drinking in the months leading up to my sister Jane leaving had, no doubt, contributed to its disappointing performance, but my sense of failure, embarrassment and guilt had a profound effect on me and I simply couldn't bear how bad I felt.

This period of time may be relatively short, but it falls into five distinct stages - pre-rehab, post-rehab, falling off the wagon, commitment to AA and finally defeat. They are all tragic in their own way because I know that I did repeatedly try incredibly hard to control my drinking by creating new rules for myself about alcohol or by giving it up completely, but in the end it just became too powerful and all-consuming.

While I naively thought that I could eventually take back control of my life, those close to me just saw someone who seemed hell bent on self-destruction, and I lost more friends during this time as I pushed everyone who didn't give up on me to the limit of their love and patience.

During the months after my business stalled and my sister Jane no longer worked with me, I increasingly used alcohol to avoid dealing with reality and to numb overwhelming feelings, but this only made things immeasurably worse. I veered erratically from despair, self-pity and fear, to arrogance and recklessness, and then back through fear, self-loathing, despair, anger, the list goes on, all fuelled by alcohol.

When I was afraid, I begged my GP for Antabuse. In despair I twice rang the police to try to get myself arrested and I decided frequently that I would be better off dead. When I was arrogant and reckless I treated my loved ones, especially Ross, with contempt and disregard, frequently drove the car drunk, ruined countless social events and was aggressive and vile to everyone from airport security staff to bus drivers.

I also ended up in hospital and had paramedics treat me at home, but I couldn't remember how or why.

This chaotic and dangerous existence, lead to me being admitted to rehab for a second time, (full details in Chapter 5), but unlike the first time, when I picked up the phone myself in desperation, this time I was very reluctant to go because I was so scared.

After spending five weeks in rehab which included missing Michael's eighteenth birthday and cancelling our family holiday, I returned home feeling like a duck out of water and very fragile, but full of resolve and determined to remain sober. I did what I had been told and I went to AA meetings, avoided triggers and promised myself and everyone close to me that I would never drink again.

This lasted for a couple of months until Christmas, when I just couldn't get the thought of alcohol out of my head. It seemed to be absolutely everywhere and so, overwhelmed by craving it, I convinced myself that a bit of secret drinking without anyone being aware wouldn't do anyone any harm - so long as no one ever found out.

To help me to achieve this, instead of drinking large bottles of wine which were difficult to hide, I turned again to spirits such as brandy and whisky which came in miniature bottles. I explained to shop assistants that they were for cooking Christmas food, never realising that only a person with a drinking problem would feel the need to justify buying miniatures.

It didn't take long for my life to completely unravel again, culminating in a very nasty accident with a kitchen mandolin, which was extremely distressing and upsetting for Ross and Michael.

Michael moved out to be with his Dad because he felt so let down after trusting me post rehab. It was his A Level year - and he basically just couldn't bear to be around me. Distraught because of this, I threw myself into AA again, this time doing it properly by getting myself a Sponsor, attending more meetings every week and working on the Twelve Steps.

As I said at the beginning, this has been incredibly difficult for me to write about because I love Michael and Ross so much and I let them down so badly.

Over the following seven months I went from feeling that I was fighting for my sobriety and my life and to get my family's respect back, (I knew that this time really was my last chance), to slowly allowing the tiny, occasional whisperings from my dark shadow to start to chip away at my resolve, distorting my memories of how bad things had been.

I slowly but surely forgot about the tear stained letters that I had written to Michael and Ross begging for their forgiveness. I forgot about the look of complete disgust on Ross' face which had only recently turned into a half smile of hope because I was spending time with my AA Sponsor and working through the Twelve Steps. I also forgot about the ache in my liver that I had felt before I went into rehab - and I started to secretly drink again.

Early 2013

There's a saying about comparison being the thief of joy and I think you could also say that comparison was the fuel of my alcoholism.

Because I felt like a complete failure after Jane left the business, I began to compare myself to my friends and peers who were successful, and I became very bitter and resentful. I hated myself for getting us into so much debt and then not achieving the success with the business that I imagined I would.

I think I knew deep down that my heavy drinking and the fact that I wasn't 'on the ball' over the previous year had definitely impacted on the business, but that didn't stop me from wallowing in self-pity and turning to increasing amounts of wine to take away feelings of guilt and regret that I was unable to handle.

I would be working and come across something that Jane had written while she worked with me and I would burst into tears and feel overwhelmed with sadness, and then drink it away. As a result, Michael temporarily moved in with his Dad, because he hated what he faced when he came home from school, which just gave me a further excuse to wallow in self-pity even more. I would cancel seeing my dog walking friends at the last minute, even though I knew in my heart that they didn't believe my excuses and they knew that something was wrong.

Something that also changed to an alarming degree was the impact that alcohol now had on my personality, which was quite scary.

Whilst alcohol had never had a positive effect on me or enhanced any of my nicer qualities in any way, it now made me very aggressive and confrontational, even with close friends who I had always tried to be on my best behaviour around.

In the January of this year, my three close university friends and I decided that we should start the year as we meant to go on, by seeing more of each other and we met up at my friend Vicky's house for drinks, laughs - a really lovely thing that normal people do with friends. I know that I had been drinking before I met them, as that was the norm for me by now, so by the time we had shared a few glasses of wine I was horribly drunk. I decided that my dear friend Paula was not giving me eye contact when she was talking and that she was deliberately ignoring me and I confronted her and caused a scene, which spoiled the whole night.

At a dinner party at another friend's house, I turned to Ross and very loudly accused our hosts of deliberately not pouring me enough wine and then burst into tears. Ross was understandably mortified and we quickly left. In both instances I felt ashamed and full of remorse the following day. I phoned everyone concerned to say that I was sorry and I was under pressure or some other feeble excuse and, because friends do, they forgave me.

However people were increasingly feeling uncomfortable around me because I could be so unpleasant and no one wants to spend an evening feeling on edge.

I found myself screaming drunk down the phone to my business bank manager, telling him it was his fault that my business wasn't doing well and I once got out of my car in the middle of the road, (over the limit), to shout at a bus driver parked at a bus stop, while the bus passengers and pedestrians looked on in horror. I was lucky I wasn't breathalysed and arrested, (although, in retrospect, that would probably have been a blessing).

I followed a woman into the supermarket who, I believed, had stolen my parking space and caused a scene, never thinking she might realise that I was drunk driving at the time.

In the end, because of the change that alcohol brought about in my personality and because I was often worried that people would suspect that I was drunk, I began to avoid talking to people all together and so I came across as cold and unfriendly.

Not long after this, Ross and I went for what was meant to be a romantic break skiing, but I started my holiday as soon as we got to the airport. Many people do this, and there's nothing wrong with having a drink or two before boarding a flight, but I hit the duty free with the speed of a whippet when he was getting a newspaper, (I'd told him I was going to the toilet). I downed several miniatures of vodka in the toilets before insisting that I had wine in the bar before we got on the plane. Once we were at our destination, I raided the alcohol cupboard of the friends who had trusted us with their skiing accommodation and hid a bottle of vodka to have when Ross wasn't looking. (Vodka now became my 'secret' drink because it achieved an effect very quickly and was easier to hide than lots of bottles of wine).

So I spent the few days we were there permanently drunk, because I was having my secret vodka and then 'legitimate' wine with Ross as well. As a result I had several really bad falls on the slopes, hitting my head and having to be picked up by strangers, and Ross genuinely did not understand why. I was such a brilliant liar and so aggressive if questioned, that poor Ross didn't know what was wrong.

Spring 2013

By now I was hiding bottles everywhere, from wellingtons to the pockets of dressing gowns, folded up in towels in the airing cupboard and in clothes in my wardrobe and also under the mattresses of the beds. I used to panic if I forgot where I had a full bottle of wine, and if I couldn't find it I sometimes even poked holes in the bottom of Ross' cans of lager, draining the contents into a bottle, so that they still looked unopened, (I'd then replace the cans and the cycle would then begin again).

My life completely revolved around buying and hiding alcohol, trying to hide the fact that I had been drinking, whilst inwardly battling with hating myself, worrying about my sanity and my health, wanting desperately to confide in someone and tell them that this was now much more serious than I had ever imagined. If we were going out I would hang back or make an excuse to go back into the house to gulp down a last drink and I also had to have frequent 'sweeps' of the house when I was alone, where I would gather together all of my empties and drive them in bin bags to different bins around where we lived. When I did manage to prepare the orders generated by the business and take them to the post office, I would buy cans of gin and tonic to hide around the house, usually drinking one on the journey home.

By this stage, alcohol consumes so much of an alcoholic's thinking, that they have room for little else. You are either congratulating yourself for not drinking, or persuading yourself that you can have a drink, or feeling guilty about lying – it is so draining and wastes so much precious energy. A horrible, constant pressure on the brain and on your sanity, it becomes unbearable.

I also started to realise that if I managed not to have a drink for a few days it made me feel really ill and so I became obsessed with reading about alcohol withdrawal and what alcoholics experience 12, 24, 48, 72 hours after having their last drink. This was to convince myself, again, that I was not an alcoholic, because I didn't experience the shakes, (for example), if I didn't drink. I was always trying to find evidence that I wasn't an alcoholic, and we all know that if you research enough, you can find evidence to prove anything! It never dawned on me that the fact that I was carrying out research in order to prove that I wasn't an alcoholic, was actually proof that I was – that and my frequent need for heartburn medication.

The reality that withdrawal was becoming a problem for me became evident in April that year when my sister Eileen celebrated her fiftieth birthday and a group of us took the 'party ferry' from Newcastle to Amsterdam. I knew I had to sober up to be around my sisters, but I hadn't expected the extreme anxiety and awful nausea that I experienced on the day that we met. I had to claim that I had severe sea sickness, and then stayed in my cabin for the overnight crossing, sending Ross to party with them.

I still felt very ill when we landed in Amsterdam and the day is a bit of a blur, but I remember feeling so alone, scared and ashamed because of the horrible secret I had. I was so relieved that Ross and I were staying on to drive to visit his sister in France, and as soon as we waved my family off I was straight into the hotel bar, justifying having a drink to Ross because I had missed out on the partying. The sense of relief that I felt having a drink again was so powerful that it took me aback, but I knew that I didn't want to stop drinking ever again after that.

I understand now that avoiding the awful withdrawal that comes with being an alcoholic is one of the things that keeps alcoholics drinking, and from that time it definitely made my drinking become more of a necessity than a choice. It wasn't that I was having awful shakes or hallucinating at that point, but the severe anxiety of withdrawal was something that I came to dread and so it began that I always felt a need to have some alcohol in my system or to remain 'topped up' so to speak, in order to avoid feeling that level of 'impending doom' anxiety.

By trying to maintain the necessary level of alcohol in my system to avoid experiencing withdrawal, I wasn't necessarily always very drunk, or even noticeably drunk to people around me. I just began to spend my waking hours in a horrible 'twilight' state and awful feeling of fuzziness and just generally feeling quite ill.

This inevitably had a further impact on my ability to run the business properly and I would often realise that I hadn't replied to important emails or sent out orders for days, and I would feel overwhelmed by the backlog of work that had mounted up.

My sister Jane would drop everything to come and help me, and she never once criticised me or told anyone. Her support at that time definitely prevented the business from collapsing completely and I am forever grateful that she was always there for me. I know that she realised that something was very wrong, but I convinced myself that my lies and excuses for not getting things done were plausible and believed.

I would frequently cancel events like walking the dog with my friends, telling them that I was busy with the business and they would often kindly offer to take our dog out with them while I 'got on with work'. Once they came back to the house and found me unconscious and half naked on the floor, (to this day I don't know why) after they had left me 'working' at my desk. I don't know how I tried to explain that particular incident away, but I do know that I was drunk for so much of the time by then, that I probably forgot about it very quickly, whereas in the past I would've been mortified for days or weeks. I can also remember my friend Vicky saying to me 'you can't do this to people Sue', when I would cancel an event with about half an hour's notice, because I simply couldn't sober up.

I also tested my friends and sisters patience by ringing them up when I was drunk, thinking that they wouldn't notice while I rambled on and I would sit up late into the night listening to music and putting embarrassing things on social media. The next day would start with deleting social media posts and frantic messaging to make sure that I hadn't upset anyone and then the whole sad cycle would begin again.

May – July 2013

Things came to head in May when I visited an old friend in Belfast for a weekend. We had worked together years before in the pharmaceutical industry and because she hadn't seen me for a long time, I looked forward to having a drunken weekend and a laugh without being judged.

Even though I knew I could happily drink a few bottles of wine with her because that is what I had always done, I still felt the need to secretly have a gulp of wine from the bottle in the fridge on both mornings before she got up or when she was in the shower, to keep me 'topped up'.

I thought that this would go unnoticed, but when we were having lunch on the Sunday before I got my flight home, she said that she knew I had a problem and that I needed to seek help, which was such a brave and loving thing to do.

I was embarrassed and adamant that she was wrong, and when I left her I felt upset and angry. I had a row with security at Belfast airport about my makeup bag containing liquids and was told that if I didn't calm down I would be escorted away. I then drank more in the bar in the departure lounge and ended up missing my flight altogether.

Ross and Michael were waiting at the other end and I knew that I would have to face the music when I eventually got home much later that night – so I got even more drunk (I thought I may as well because I was in trouble anyway).

My run in with airport security and missing my flight was enough to frighten me into promising that I would get help - again. I had become a virtual stranger now to Michael, who was spending most of his time at his Dad's and he never brought friends home anymore because I had become an embarrassment to him.

I sobbed at the GP surgery and begged for Antabuse, but they said that it is too dangerous a drug to prescribe for someone like me. Instead I was offered a drug called Acamprosate. This was completely inappropriate because it should only be prescribed for people who have already stopped drinking, to prevent future urges to drink. I was then referred to a local NHS alcohol service and began to go for counselling.

Deep down I was terrified to give up alcohol completely, so I told Ross that I was working with my counsellor to address my issues and to learn how to drink in moderation. He did not question this because he trusted me, partly because I also convinced him that it would be dangerous for me to give up alcohol completely because of the risk of seizure (something that I had read about withdrawal was now a useful piece of information to stop him from challenging me. The seizures sometimes experienced by chronic alcoholics when they suddenly stop drinking can be fatal). When I went to see my counsellor I again always dressed smartly and said what they wanted to hear, all the while lying that I had given up drinking.

I hated myself so much by this time and was terrified of what I was turning into. Part of me wanted to cry and reach out to people to help, but then I'd realise that I couldn't imagine not being able to drink.

Anyone who is constantly 'topped up' with alcohol is obviously incapable of leading a secret life for any prolonged period of time, because you would need your wits permanently about you for that. Because of this I would frequently slip up and forget how much I had secretly been drinking and then appear so very obviously drunk to everyone, when they had believed that I was not drinking. This was when I started to actually truly believe that I had the power to 'drink myself sober'. This is no exaggeration, even though it sounds unbelievable.

If I'd accidentally had more to drink when Ross was at work than I had intended to, I honestly believed that if I had a bit more to drink I would somehow sober up. Insane behaviour, but I began to do this more and more and would increasingly crawl to bed and pass out during the day. Suddenly this became the norm and our home life became a twilight zone with me sleeping when I should've been there for my husband and son.

As they always say in AA rooms, books on alcoholism and in rehab - alcoholism is not just about the alcoholic, it is a 'disease' of the whole family and our family life began to disintegrate. I still had days where I would function and work on my business and cook a meal, but my drinking was now just a fact of life and Ross and Michael just adapted to it and got on with their own lives. I pretended that the counselling was a waste of time and of no help to me and Ross didn't try to argue with me. He was at the end of his patience and so I tried to save my massive drinking blowouts for when he was away with work, so that he would detest me a little less, but this didn't always go to plan.

When I was functioning I would panic and try to create new rules. I had noticed a nagging dull ache in my liver and so I would try to give up alcohol. I would count the hours since I had had a drink, (12, 24, 48, 72 hours), and feel relieved and pleased with myself, only for the anxiety and stomach cramps to start, which would only go away if I had a drink.

Sometimes I would battle through this withdrawal and have a few days off to manically catch up with outstanding business issues, check in with my friends and family and try to do housework, only to eventually convince myself that this proved that I wasn't an alcoholic after all. I would often try different tactics to stop myself from drinking, such as imagining that it was someone who didn't like me or whom I was jealous of, offering me a drink to sabotage my life, or I would imagine that Michael could see me reaching for the bottle, but I always eventually gave in and got that huge rush of relief after the first gulp.

Unbelievably, I was still involved with the charity and was now on their committee to organise the annual ball which was due to take place in September. I had already managed to persuade my Radio DJ friend from the 'Angels of The North' to host the evening for the charity, so I turned up for a couple of meetings on the planning committee worse for wear, but then I then made excuses that the business was so busy that I couldn't commit to regular meetings, and didn't want to keep letting them down. To divert their attention from my glazed eyes and also to make myself feel better about letting them down, I offered for my tiny business to sponsor the printing for the ball- a grand gesture and deliberate attempt at a smokescreen, but something that the business could not even afford. I also attended one of their lunchtime fundraisers with my friend Gayle, who ended up having to phone Ross to help me home because I had got so drunk - even though we'd only been listening to a talk on arts and crafts.

In reality I just didn't want to be around people regularly in case they realised that I'd been drinking and gradually I stopped making plans with anyone, because I couldn't guarantee that I would even manage to turn up, or to turn up sober. I cancelled friends visiting us and I let Ross down many times when he had bought us tickets to see something.

One event that I had signed up for was to climb Ben Nevis in July that year, to raise money for the charity. This was partly to prove, yet again, that I wasn't an alcoholic, because if I was, there would be no way that I could complete such a physical challenge. I somehow completed the climb and Ross and Michael met me back in Glasgow. They probably thought to themselves that maybe I was finally getting a grip on things because of this achievement.

Just after this, Ross and I went for a long weekend to Prague, which he had arranged months before as a special treat. This was honestly one of the happiest times we had shared together for a long time. I stuck to drinking beer instead of bottles of wine and didn't get hideously drunk, just generally 'topped up'. I wasn't aggressive or emotional and we both thought that the worst was over and that I had turned a corner.

Unfortunately, we were wrong.

August 2013

The unfathomable thing about alcohol is the relentless and brutal games that it plays with your head and your life. You're a crazy drunk one minute and full of remorse the next, then you manage sobriety or controlled drinking for a while, until you think you're on top of it, then it throws you back down, knocks the stuffing out of you and does a body slam just to make sure you know it's in charge. August 2013 was that time for me.

I had thought that my behaviour couldn't get any more out of control than the close shave with security in Belfast airport. I believed that I would never allow myself to let Michael and Ross down again in the way I had been doing for the last nine months or so, but in August I surpassed even my darkest fears as to where alcohol would take me.

As you are aware by now, I have come to regard alcoholism as a kind of evil entity that only wants to destroy the alcoholic and cruelly hurt those around them and so this continued to happen for me.

After our lovely break in Prague I arrived home full of hope that I could put the difficult months behind me and rebuild my relationship with Michael, as well as working at getting my business back on track and even, hopefully, gain some self-respect and eventually the respect of my friends and family. So the events of the next few weeks honestly came out of absolutely nowhere and I still can't make sense of what happened, even now.

Within days of getting home I felt overwhelmed by guilt, shame and bitterness again, feeling sorry for myself and desperate for a drink. Ross had to get on with his job and couldn't babysit me 24/7, and I somehow found myself sitting in the car at a cemetery near our house, drinking miniatures of wine and sobbing - wishing that I was dead.

I hated what I had become and couldn't see a way out any more, and the alcohol fuelled my feelings of failure and self-loathing. In some sort of pathetic cry for help, I called the police to tell them that I was drink driving, but I lost my nerve and hung up after crying to the operator that I was very sorry. I did this a second time and then sobbed in the driving seat and drank some more wine.

I didn't realise that the call handler had traced my number to our house and Ross quickly had a visit from the police who asked him what was going on. He managed to convince them that we'd had a row and that I had then gone off, not drunk, but very upset. He had to apologise profusely for wasting their time and he was completely shaken and shocked by their visit because he had no idea what was going on.

After ringing my phone for ages because I had passed out, he managed to speak to me and finally tracked me down, walking to the cemetery and driving me home. He was furious, but I was so out of it and unable to even stand, that I just had to go to bed to sleep it off. Obviously I was full of remorse the next day, but I felt so ill that the main thing on my mind was having another drink to feel better.

Ross had to go away for a couple of days but Michael had moved back in with us at that time, so I tried to secretly drink without Michael knowing, (Ross had not told him about the cemetery). On the afternoon of the day that I was meant to pick Ross up from the airport, I found myself feeling much more drunk than I had intended, so my 'drinking myself sober' mentality kicked in. I was convinced that if I had a bit more wine I would appear more sober to Michael - my mind really was that messed up.

Even though driving whilst over the limit was something, I had frequently done before, I knew I had now gone way beyond the limits that I had somehow enforced on myself and that I couldn't possibly drive the car to the airport. However, to 'convince' Michael that I hadn't been drinking, I pretended to go to the airport and drove my car up a little dirt track into some woods next to our house.

Sitting drunk again in my parked up car, the enormity of my problem and an overwhelming fear hit me, but I was so drunk that everything was distorted in my head and I felt completely out of control. I rang the police again and said that I was a drink driver who needed to be arrested - and then fell asleep.

The police duly arrived at the house and when Michael saw them he thought I must have had an accident. Ross arrived at the airport and when he realised that I wasn't there to pick him up, he had a sick feeling that something awful had happened. Then, when his taxi arrived at our house and he saw two police cars outside, he naturally feared the worst. Both Ross and Michael thought that I was dead, when I was selfishly and unforgivably sleeping in my car in the woods next to our house, drunk.

The police started to search the area and as they did so, I woke up and staggered down to the house. I can't even remember getting home, but Ross told me that I was sobbing and saying I was sorry as we all stood in the kitchen, and he told the police I was going through the menopause and that my emotions had become very unstable. One of the female officers wanted to arrest me, but another officer pointed out that I hadn't driven the car on a public highway, so they left us, very angry that their time had been wasted by a sad, middle aged drunk.

How Michael and Ross must have felt standing in the kitchen of the house, looking at me in such a state after thinking that I was dead I will never know, but I know that they hated the person that I now was. Yet again I was full of remorse but again Michael couldn't bear to be around me and moved out. Even that wasn't enough to stop me drinking by then and when Ross was at work I gulped down vodka like I drank wine, straight out of the bottle. Not surprisingly, I almost poisoned myself, because if I had ever drunk spirits in the past, it had been from miniature bottles, just to keep me 'topped up'.

Twice, over the next two weeks, Ross found me unconscious on the floor. The first time he called Paramedics to the house and they satisfied themselves that I hadn't taken any pills on top of the vodka, and then they left me at home to sleep it off. The first I knew of this was when I woke up the next day and asked Ross what the 'sticky stuff' on my chest was and he flatly told me that it was from the pads that the paramedics had stuck on my skin when they were monitoring my heart – he was so disgusted and angry. I couldn't remember anything about it and felt deeply ashamed for wasting their time and also terrified.

All this time, Ross never told my family or friends about how bad things had become out of a sense of loyalty to me and also in the hope that I could get back to the Sue that he had fallen in love with – I suppose that admitting what was going on in our lives to other people would make it 'real', and he was at a total loss as to how to deal with my behaviour.

Ross had to cope with all of this whilst continuing to work in his very demanding job every day, and he somehow managed to do that. No one should be put in that position or have to deal with living like that, and I know he struggled for a long time with his feelings towards me and was so fed up with me that he wanted to leave.

However, the cat was finally let out of the bag the second time in as many days that Ross found me unconscious at home, and I think that this came as an enormous relief to him, because the burden of the secret eventually just became too much to bear. This second time, before I gulped down half a bottle of vodka in one go and passed out, I had sent a message to some family and friends saying that I was a horrible person and they would be better off if I wasn't around. Yet again, unforgivably selfish behaviour, more so because I passed out just after sending it, so I was completely unaware of the frantic texts and calls from people who were alarmed and worried by what they had read.

Again Ross became so frightened when he couldn't rouse me at all that he thought I might have also taken some pills. I eventually woke up much later in hospital connected to a drip, with Ross looking ashen sitting next to the bed.

While we were at the hospital my sisters Jane and Eileen, who had read my text, had rushed to the house after they had been unable to contact me or Ross. They too thought that I was dead and were still at the house when I was discharged from hospital and driven home by Ross. There was no lying my way out of it this time or any possibility that Ross would cover for me. I was actually too ill to explain what had been going on to Eileen and Jane and so I left Ross downstairs to fill them in.

I obviously had no problem going to sleep or falling unconscious, but when I woke up the next day with that overwhelming anxiety and sense of doom that all alcoholics know, I knew that I just couldn't go on like this any longer – it was as if I was trying to kill myself with vodka, without actually wanting to die.

In desperation and at the end of his tether, Ross had called Mark's mother for help. She was extremely kind and generous and she arranged for me to go into rehab. It was incredibly difficult for Ross and very brave, but he had nowhere left to turn and felt completely helpless.

When he told me, instead of feeling gratitude or relief, I only felt fear and panic - fear about not being able to drink ever again and panic about what everyone would think of me. I had taken for granted that my secret was safe with Ross, and I had treated him so badly and had never once given serious thought to the impact that all of this was having on him. Part of me wanted to say 'you've got this all wrong, it was just a one off and I'm not really that bad. I can change, I promise…….' – but the other part of me knew that if I didn't go, I would lose everyone and almost certainly end up dead.

September 2013 - January 2014

I tried to delay going into rehab for three reasons. We would miss Michael's eighteenth birthday, we had a two week holiday booked and were meant to travel in a few days, and I would also miss the charity ball that I had, (partly), helped to organise. However, Michael said that the best birthday present I could give to him would be to come back sober and Ross immediately cancelled our holiday - something that he had worked so hard for and needed more than most.

In a panic, I pleaded to delay and said that I would need recovery time before I could leave for rehab in order to sober up. Deep down this was really intended to give me more drinking time because I was literally terrified of not being able to drink ever again.

Understandably and predictably, no one was interested in what I had to say, and so on September 6th 2013 I was packed off to rehab and I cried the whole way there.

Because the fact that rehab did not work for me is one of the main reasons for writing this book, (that and my failed attempts at AA), and my experiences there require a whole chapter, I have devoted all of Chapter 5 to talk about my two experiences in rehab. However what I want to make clear here is that, although I was initially reluctant to go, once I was there and had fully sobered up, I really did give it my all and tried very hard, and I was determined that I would never drink again once I left.

As I cover in Chapter 5, during the five weeks that I spent in the second rehab, I did learn a lot about myself and alcoholism, and I also met some brilliant people. One of the overwhelming feelings that I experienced throughout my time in there was humility, because of the overwhelming pure love and support that I received from Ross, Michael and my family and friends, even after everything that I had put them through.

I felt incredibly lucky that I was being given this chance because of the generosity of Mark's Mum, (as well as very lucky that my excessive drinking had not caused any obvious physical damage), and when Ross came to pick me up in the middle of October, I was a different person. I felt very sheepish and nervous, but hopeful that I could make amends to him and Michael, and I was determined to create a normal home life for us again, without alcohol.

Back at home, I felt like a duck out of water. Although rehab prepares you for moving back home and coping mechanisms for a life without alcohol, and I did all of the things that I had been told to do, like going to AA meetings, avoiding triggers, avoiding isolating myself etc., I was ultimately relying on my own willpower and avoidance tactics, and I found it increasingly difficult. What I hadn't anticipated or been prepared for was just how awkward and exposed I felt, and it was as if I was learning to be a human being all over again. I was full of paranoia and insecurity, thinking that everyone was whispering about me and convincing myself that they were watching to see if I was shaking or slurring or sneaking off for a drink. To be fair, if they were thinking that who could blame them, but it made me uptight and self-conscious and I felt like nothing was real.

I tried desperately hard to be 'normal' whilst at the same time trying to encourage Ross and Michael to talk about how they felt – I think I just wanted them to tell me what a selfish cow I had been and to get it off their chests. This was unfair of me and I expected too much of them, because they just wanted normality, routine and a wife and mother who was predictable and reliable - not endless psychoanalysis with outpourings of contrition and remorse.

Outside of our home life, when I was with other people, I felt out of my depth and anxious. I was frequently on the defensive because I was ashamed about my past behaviour and felt exposed and completely out of my comfort zone, all the while battling the urge to drink because I believed alcohol would take away this awkwardness and give me back my 'normality' and confidence and my dark shadow whispered exactly that. By the time Christmas came, I felt as if I was hanging on to sobriety by my fingernails and I was feeling beaten down, as if my willpower was slowly slipping away and getting weaker.

I shared this at AA, but I felt that I couldn't tell anyone close to me because I imagined the groans of 'here we go again' and so I kept this raging battle going on inside me from everyone. I was frightened to admit just how difficult I was finding things and what a struggle it was for me not to pick up a drink, but at the same time, I wanted our lives to be normal again. I didn't want Ross to miss out on things because I wasn't drinking, so I accepted invitations to Christmas events and told him I would be fine. This was also because I didn't want anyone else to think that I had 'changed'.

However when I was around other people I felt clumsy, stiff, (I couldn't dance for the life of me!), and on edge, because I thought that I was boring. These feelings were compounded when one of our 'couple' friends suddenly dropped us from their lives completely, because they felt uncomfortable about me going to rehab and not being able to drink socially any more.

I can see now that it was such early days in my sobriety and that all of these feelings were completely normal and I was expecting too much. Anyone with experience of alcoholism knows that giving up is the easy part and it's staying sober and not picking up a drink again, that's incredibly difficult. It all eventually became too much for me and my dark shadow's whispering grew louder and more insistent. I stupidly went shopping to buy alcohol as a Christmas gift for someone and I made the insane decision to go into a wine shop, where I was surrounded by easy to hide miniatures. 'Just one' the dark shadow whispered.......

January 2014 - August 2014

The fact that I picked up a drink and threw the love, support and trust of Michael and Ross back in their faces makes me feel sick even today. That voice inside your head, which every alcoholic knows, makes you believe that it will be different this time.

Again I managed to convince myself that I wasn't as bad as people made out, the people I'd met in rehab and AA were far worse than me, I wouldn't ever let it get out of hand again because I'd learned my lesson, and if people didn't know that I was drinking it wouldn't do any harm......

Unbelievable and unforgivably selfish I know, but that's how alcohol works. I actually convinced myself that the hospital and police incidents had been extreme reactions to stressful events, that they would never be repeated and I could now drink safely - in secret.

In the New Year I had booked a tiny, romantic cottage for Ross' Birthday for a couple of days, but ruined the entire break by smuggling brandy in my bag. I was drunk before we even got to the cottage and Ross snapped, he'd had enough and he told me that he just couldn't take any more. Yet again I promised that it wouldn't happen again, and probably had a week or so of trying not to be visibly drunk around Ross and Michael, but in the middle of January, everything came crashing down once more.

They say that when and alcoholic starts drinking again after a period of sobriety, they don't just pick off where they left off, they surpass however hellish it was before and the effects of the alcohol on the person are even more extreme. This is certainly true of my own experience. Before I knew it, I was back to where I had been during the previous summer.

My drinking was out of control, but on this particular day I had miscalculated how much I had been drinking, which meant I then tried to drink myself sober, which predictably didn't work. So, in order to create a smoke screen to divert Ross and Michael's attention from the fact that I was drunk, I decided that it would be a good idea to cook something special, because I believed that they would conclude that I couldn't possibly be drunk if I had cooked something nice. That is how my insane alcoholic mind worked.

I decided to make dauphinoise potatoes, which meant using the razor sharp mandolin to slice the potatoes thinly. I was so drunk by this time that I cannot remember slicing the end of my little finger off or passing out in bed, but Ross arrived home to a kitchen covered in blood and Michael in his room, upset and angry.

Ross had to go away on a work trip the following day and when I woke up and saw the blood stained bandage on my finger he flatly said, 'that's the least of your worries'. He had rung my friend Vicky the night before and asked if she could take me to her house to stay for a few days - Michael had had enough and was moving out again, and Ross was looking forward to a few days away from me, when he could do some serious thinking about our future.

Vicky arrived at 7am, Ross and Michael left the house without another word and I can remember being in total shock. How had I gone from being sober after rehab, to a situation where Ross and Michael were potentially out of my life for good? Vicky rang my dog-walking friend who was also a nurse, to check out my finger. Afterwards I told Vicky that I would follow her to her house in my car, hoping that I could secretly stock up on alcohol on the way because I could not bear the thought of sobering up and having to face what I had done. Thankfully she was having none of it because she knew exactly what my plans were, and she drove us both to her house.

I was still drunk by the time we arrived at her home. She ran me a bath and then I went to bed to sleep it off. I honestly didn't want to wake up and wished I was dead. When I did wake up the next day I had the shakes and felt sick, but I couldn't have a drink and so then the awful, overwhelming anxiety started.

I was frantic and scared, and terrified that I had lost Ross and Michael and didn't know where to put myself. Vicky was amazing and was kinder to me than I deserved. She gave me a notebook and said that I couldn't change what had happened, but I could start planning for how I was going to get better and fix things. She listened to me sob about being afraid to die and how I couldn't bear to lose my son and my husband. She also drove me to an AA meeting and stayed with me while I just cried. She even had to deal with being gently chastised by the people at the meeting, because she wasn't an alcoholic herself and shouldn't have been there.

For the whole time that I was at her house, I tried to ring Michael and sent messages to him, but he wouldn't answer. I wrote notes to him, trying to explain how I felt in the hope that I could show them to him one day. I did speak on the phone to Ross and promised him that I would do AA properly this time, I would get myself a Sponsor and work the Twelve Steps, like I should've done before. I swore on my life that I would change and begged to be given another chance, and Ross told me that he still loved me and would help me.

I rang AA in desperation, because I realised that if I failed to stay sober this time, there really was no hope left and no more options left for me. A lovely lady met me for a coffee. She would eventually become my Sponsor, (Chapter 6 is devoted to AA), and she agreed to take me to meetings – it can be quite daunting turning up on your own.

This was my last chance to get sober and I knew that if I didn't, not only would I lose Ross and Michael altogether, but I would die. I knew then that I was in the grip of something that I had completely underestimated, that it was destroying me, and I was so afraid.

Michael was still out of my life, and I understood that the only way he would want to know me again would be if I was sober – and he had believed that I was sober after rehab. It was his A Level year and I didn't want to mess his life up anymore, so I used my notebook from Vicky to plan my weekly timetable of AA meetings as well as SMART Therapy sessions – a relatively new approach then, but I was desperate to try anything.

I talk about my experiences with AA in detail in Chapter 6, but I'll confirm here that I did go to meetings several times a week and threw myself wholeheartedly into working through the Twelve Steps properly with my Sponsor. I met her outside of our time in meetings and made friends with people from the group, something that I hadn't done before. This lasted for months – longer than my sobriety after rehab, but by the summer, the little voice that had started as a whisper began to get louder and louder, again lying to me that I wasn't as bad as the other alcoholics in AA, and that I had proved I was 'cured' because I had been sober for a while.

And now comparison, after being the fuel of my alcoholism in the beginning, was to become the thief of my hard fought sobriety, because I was comparing myself to other alcoholics, and slowly coming to the conclusion that maybe I wasn't that bad after all……….

At this point, I want to share some of the desperate notes that I wrote, but never sent, to Michael and Ross, and also to myself, after I picked up a drink a few months after my second stint in rehab –

'Darling Michael. I am sitting at Vicky's aching for you. To talk to you, to cuddle you. I didn't think of that yesterday. All I felt was selfish. I now feel so alone and frightened that I have lost you. I feel so totally bereft. I love you more than anything – how could I even think of having a drink? My stomach is churning and my head feels like it will explode with the feelings of total shame and sadness that I have. I am so, so sorry and I can't bear to know that I have hurt you and let you down again. I want to beat this horrible disease and I know that I can. Please forgive me my darling boy. I am so frightened.'

'Drink is ruining my whole life. Please, please God help me. I don't want to feel like this ever again and I don't want to lose Ross and Michael.'

'Darling Ross. I feel so frightened and I am so sorry. Please forgive me.'

'Avoid situations where people are drinking – it is not ok and I am not ok when I am there. I get jealous of people drinking, so I must avoid it. Go to regular meetings – more than three per week. Find a sponsor and arrange SMART meetings. This is worse than ever and I am so, so frightened and I cannot do this on my own. I am treating my alcoholism as if it is a terminal illness. AA and SMART are the medicine that I need to take. If I take them regularly every week I won't die – it's as simple as that. Also, I need to stop comparing my life to others.'

'Feeling sad and wretched as usual. Please, please God, help me to beat this curse. What did I ever do to feel so crap. This isn't how I saw my life panning out and this is no way to live.'

'Being an alcoholic is a fucking curse and I hate it and hate me at the moment.'

'Susan, please read this if you are ever tempted to drink. It never changes – in fact it always gets worse. You are feeling wretched and desperate and physically very ill. You cannot drink safely. Don't do it. Cravings pass.'

I have shared those very private notes because even after writing them and then going to AA for months, alcohol won and I started to drink secretly again. This is hard to believe when I had been so sorry and so desperate, but by then my dark shadow was much more powerful than any willpower I had within me and I didn't stand a chance.

Chapter 4

Counselling, Hypnotherapy and Other Treatments

Writing this book has been incredibly challenging for me, because it has brought back some very raw emotions that are so powerful they can still make me weep. The challenge I have faced with this chapter is to prevent myself from getting carried away on a rant. Firstly when I reflect upon the time and money that I wasted over the years on treatments that didn't work, from people who I feel may have taken advantage of the desperate state I found myself in. I like to believe that the majority of people are fundamentally decent human beings, and that those who are drawn to a profession which involves helping others begin from a good place in their heart. But some people did say that they could help me when they shouldn't have.

Secondly, because of the frustration that I feel about what I see as the blinkered and old fashioned approach that many healthcare professionals still take when dealing with an alcoholic, because they still assume that counselling, AA and rehab should work for anyone who genuinely wants to stop drinking.

There are a lot of people out there making a lot of money out of alcoholics, (or their families or friends), by claiming that that they can help the person get back to being a 'social drinker' or to stop them from drinking completely. However if we look below the surface, it is very difficult to establish actual concrete success rates, and this applies to AA and rehab also.

In my experience, there is still a great deal of stigma surrounding alcoholism that has resulted in a naïve and narrow minded approach as to how to best deal with a person who is struggling with alcohol, especially when they present to their GP, whether that be in the early stages when their drinking is becoming a problem, or when they are further down the alcoholic spiral.

I do appreciate that, from an NHS point of view, resources are very limited and alcoholism comes way down the list of priorities, including in the training of new doctors. However, the burden that the consequences of excessive drinking is placing on the NHS is huge, whether that be from accidents or serious alcohol related illnesses, so I think that the approach to patients presenting with alcohol problems is in need of a long overdue overhaul.

Consequently, during the several visits I made to different GP's over the years, when I was concerned about my drinking, I was offered counselling or advised to attend AA meetings as well as being directed to local alcohol services, which mainly involved counselling and latterly SMART Therapy.

More than once when I visited a GP with concerns about my drinking, I was offered drugs such as Acamprosate and Valium, intended to be used when someone is withdrawing from alcohol, (to deal with the horrible anxiety and prevent cravings), which illustrates a lack of understanding as to where these drugs fit, because I couldn't stop drinking, so was not at the stage where they would be useful.

So several times I, like many other people with alcohol problems, tried the options available to me through the NHS as well as spending my own, (and other people's) money on hypnotherapists, counselling and rehab. I know that I am in no way unique and my experiences must echo those of many others, and this fills me with despair.

When an alcoholic picks up the phone to someone or some organisation who they understand is able to help them to beat their addiction, they are invariably desperate - which can leave them vulnerable and open to being exploited. I know that alcoholics are not the only group of people who willingly part with their money when they are in turmoil, trusting that a stranger will miraculously fix their problems, but this is an account of my experiences with alcohol, and the many times I took a massive 'leap of faith' with a practitioner I had found on the internet, or a counsellor I was referred to by a GP.

I want people to understand the lengths that I would go to in order to 'exorcise' the alcoholism from myself and be normal again.

Sadly, like many others who find themselves in the same position that I was, I instantly blamed myself when counselling, hypnotherapy, AA etc. didn't work - and I know that those around me blamed me too. This is because we all assume that these traditional approaches to the treatment of alcoholism will work if you really want them to and that, because they are overseen by 'experts', it follows that if an alcoholic picks up a drink after having the benefit of this expertise, it must be the alcoholic who is to blame, perhaps because they have not tried hard enough or haven't done what they were told.

When I felt that I had failed, it was completely natural for me to immediately take all of the blame, and then wallow in self-pity, feel hopeless and helpless and give up – which I did many times - and then I would drink even more.

One thing that I know for certain about myself, which is no doubt true of many other people too, is that I approached each new treatment with absolute trust, and an all-consuming determination to make it work. I always had a real sense of relief and optimism when I found someone new on the internet or I was referred to a new counsellor or treatment programme by my GP. I always believed that this time I was going to beat it and that this person or organisation had all of the answers - I always felt total unwavering and heart-breaking hope.

It is also very important that I stress that in no way do I consider myself an expert in any of the treatments I am going to talk about. However, I know for sure that I am definitely an expert at being an alcoholic and at trying very hard to get sober.

Counselling

I have talked and talked and talked to different counsellors and experts over the years about my drinking, my past, my feelings and my relationships, initially attempting to control my drinking and then, ultimately, trying to stop drinking completely.

As I have stressed, I am not an expert on counselling and I know there are many situations where seeing a counsellor can really help a person to deal with life's challenges, help them to make sense of their behaviour and turn their life around.

Counselling is essential for many people who really do benefit from talking through and making sense of events in their life, and the impact those events might be having on their emotions, behaviour, relationships etc. There is a much better understanding now of conditions such as PTSD, the impact that events can have on an individual, and how to help these people move through anxiety, fear, grief…. etc.

I have met many, many alcoholics over the years and they all have some idea as to why they might have become an alcoholic, whether that be abuse or trauma as a child, bullying at school, heartbreak, bereavement….. it could be anything. Alcoholics are all individuals with thousands of stories to tell, but they all have the same very urgent issue – they need to control their drinking or stop drinking altogether, fast. One thing about alcoholism that is certain is that it is progressive. I believe that I wasted a lot of time trawling through ancient history over long periods of time, as my alcoholism silently worked away at me in the background and increasingly took hold of me and took over my life.

Typically, my counselling sessions took place weekly, especially when they were through the NHS. This meant that it was a very drawn out and slow process, whilst my alcoholism was progressing with the sole aim of taking over my life and destroying it. Counselling can often unearth painful memories and troubling feelings that are difficult to deal with, and when you do that to a person who has problems controlling their consumption of a known depressant, it doesn't take a rocket scientist to work out that this could potentially do more harm than good.

My personal experiences with counselling have been varied, but they all typically involved me talking about my past, how my drinking had impacted or was impacting those around me and my thoughts about myself.

Afterwards, I often felt worse, more wretched about what my drinking was doing to my life and the people I love, and ashamed about the past. I was almost left with more questions than I had before and no answers, which would be fine if I had the luxury of time to sort through these issues, but I was still drinking and making things worse, stuck in a vicious circle.

I need to stress very strongly that I understand that there are many mental health issues that could not be treated without counselling. I know that there are situations where counselling is a lifeline to people, and there is a very real need to talk things through instead of bottling them up. However I firmly believe, based on my own experience, that alcoholism is not one of these.

Where alcoholism is concerned, I firmly believe that there is a real and urgent need to just stop the person from drinking – it's as simple as that. Once a person is no longer drinking, they may well benefit from counselling sessions, but when alcohol has taken hold of a person and they are still drinking I think that talking is, quite frankly, futile. In my opinion, the most pressing issue is to remove alcohol from the equation as quickly as possible and I will stick my neck out and say that I believe that counselling alone does not help alcoholics to do this – it certainly did not help me.

Hypnotherapy

Before I came to the end of the line with my alcoholic journey, I had spent a couple of thousand pounds on five different hypnotherapists in different parts of the country, in an attempt to control my drinking or stop drinking completely.

As I said before, there are many people out there who are happy to take the money of a desperate alcoholic, and each time I contacted these people, it was because I was in a truly hopeless place, practically begging for help. What I now know is that alcoholism is such a notoriously difficult condition to deal with, that many hypnotherapists admit they will not attempt to help an alcoholic at all because the chances of success are so small.

Looking back at my experiences with hypnotherapy, only one of the five hypnotherapists that I saw actually stated on their website that they could help with alcoholism, with the others reassuring me that they could help me only when I contacted them to make enquiries about alcoholism.

As with many things in life, hindsight is a great thing, but when you so badly want to fix the mess you're making of your life, you will do absolutely anything, and I put my faith whole heartedly into the hands of a variety of hypnotherapists. Three of the five were, I admit, well-meaning enough but completely out of their depth and, I believe, should never have claimed that they could help me to stop drinking. They were competent hypnotherapists in other areas I am sure. I easily 'went under' hypnosis into a very relaxed state for each of them, and also I felt good when I left.

The problem was, that after maybe a couple of days of not drinking, which I'm sure was down to my own determination to prove that it had worked and I had not wasted our money, I reverted back to my old ways very quickly and immediately blamed myself for being weak and pathetic, rather than exploring the possibility that alcoholism is not the in same league as giving up smoking, overcoming a fear of flying or a spider phobia, which traditional hypnotherapy can very successfully 'cure'.

The fourth hypnotherapy session was doomed from the moment I sat down in front of the female hypnotherapist, having explained to her on the telephone that I needed to give up alcohol. She looked me up and down and said, 'I can see that the alcohol you are drinking is settling around your tummy as fat. Imagine how good you'll feel shifting that'. After that I didn't feel very relaxed at all, rather I was quite humiliated.

She somehow persuaded me to go back for a second session, but she became quite angry when I arrived and she asked me if I had had a drink since seeing her the week before. I was completely honest and told her that I had been to the local Loch Fyne restaurant and had some oysters, and you can't have oysters without white wine can you? (I had convinced Ross that this hypnotherapist was helping me to cut down on my drinking rather than give up completely and that she was very good. That was how I had managed to persuade him that I could have the wine at the restaurant).

I didn't go back to her after the second session, partly because she spent a good deal of the time explaining how the 'law of attraction' had made her very wealthy after she had visualised cheques flying through her letterbox, but mainly because I knew then that she just wasn't able to help me and that I had sadly wasted almost two hundred pounds on seeing her. Again I felt like a failure and a fool, and I also felt incredibly guilty about wasting our money.

Not one of the first four hypnotherapists spent any time getting to know me or asked about my problem in any detail, (I do not mean this in a 'counselling' way, I mean that they didn't ask for any basic background information, around which they could tailor our session).

Their approaches varied from explaining about the layers of an onion to attaching a pulse monitor to my finger, but they all seemed to use a generic script which could easily be found and printed off after an online search.

Probably the worst and most worrying hypnotherapy session I had, was with a man who I had to travel a significant distance to see. His website stated categorically that he had had a great deal of success in treating alcoholics and helping them to quit drinking completely and permanently - perfect I thought. This was during a period where I felt I needed to give up drinking altogether rather than just cut down on my alcohol consumption and I was very emotional when I contacted him. I had also looked at the testimonials on his website, and I was so confident that this was the man who could finally help me that when he told me the treatment for my alcoholism would set me back over one thousand pounds, it didn't deter me in the slightest and only seemed to make his claims even more believable. I can remember wishing that I could just see him there and then, rather than having to wait a couple of weeks for an appointment, and I willingly paid half the money up front, over the phone.

I booked into a hotel the evening before I was due to see him and I can only thank God that my good friend Karen, who I had been a Hospital Rep with all those years ago, and who is still a close friend, still worked in that part of the country. I met her for a coffee that morning and we had a very honest chat about how worried she'd been when she'd last seen me, after I'd gotten horribly drunk and been particularly hostile to Ross in front of her and her husband. Karen had known me for years and knew that I had always liked to get drunk, but she admitted that I wasn't really 'fun' anymore, which was very brave of her to say.

I asked her to come with me to the therapist's home, where I had my appointment, so that someone who cared about me knew where I was and could be sure that I left his house in one piece, and thankfully she also came inside with me. When we arrived the first thing that he wanted me to do was pay the balance for my treatment, which I thought was fair enough and I got my cheque book out, (I thought that if it didn't work I could cancel the cheque). He insisted that I used my debit card and explained that he had a card machine and I can remember being a bit disappointed because he didn't seem very 'caring'.

Once the awkward payment bit was over with, he explained that part of the treatment involved a tiny amount of electricity passing through me. He recommended that I take some Valium before we started, which he took from his drawer, so that I was relaxed for the rest of the session - he said that this would make the whole process more successful. I have to admit that I was more than happy to take the Valium, because I would've done anything that he said in order to make this work. Karen had different ideas however and very firmly told him - and me - that I wouldn't be taking any Valium and asked me if I was absolutely sure that I wanted to go ahead with the session. After the therapist and I had reassured her that I would be fine and Valium free Karen left, but asked me to contact her as soon as I was finished.

When I had made myself comfortable in the big, relaxing seat, he wheeled out what looked like a Van De Graaff Generator, (which I remembered from Physics lessons in school) and asked me to place my hand on top of it. At the same time, he placed a necklace around my neck, saying it would 'store' whatever positive energy it was that was generated during the session and that this would stop me from drinking in the future. It all sounds completely insane now, but I was so sure that his strange methods were going to fix me.

There was an element of hypnosis involved, as well as the 'putting my hand on the silver 'orb'' part, and I left his place after a couple of hours feeling a bit silly but hopeful. I then drove the two hundred or so miles back home.

Sadly, and maybe predictably, I had wasted our money again, only this time it was a lot of money to us. This meant that I had to pretend that it had worked in terms of controlling my drinking which, in my head, made it more necessary for me to hide the majority of my drinking from Ross and Michael. In reality I began drinking again almost immediately, using the fact that I felt such a fool to justify needing alcohol again.

SMART Therapy

SMART therapy was suggested by my GP but, unfortunately, it was totally inappropriate for me and for that reason I think that my personal experiences with SMART will not do it justice. In fairness, the SMART therapy that I attended was run by people who were trained professionals and qualified to deal with addiction, unlike some of the other people I have encountered, and this approach to treatment was in its infancy at the time.

When I attended SMART therapy, we discussed how I was using alcohol as a coping mechanism or crutch, and they described my problem drinking as more of a habit than a disease, which could be managed in a way that would allow me to drink again in moderation, as opposed to becoming completely abstinent.

This can only be described as music to my alcoholic ears.

I used my new SMART information to convince myself and everyone around me that my alcoholic 'episodes' had been a reaction to events that I could not cope with, and that I didn't need to give up drinking alcohol completely. I think SMART therapy might work for some people who are drinking to excess, but it was completely unsuitable for me in my situation, and I know that I used it to persuade others to allow me to get back to 'normal' drinking, and to reassure them that I wasn't an out of control alcoholic.

I did try various other things over the years in a bid to 'cure' myself including acupuncture and having crystals swung over me. I would do countless deals with God, begging for help, and even though it had been years since I'd attended church, I also sought the help of a priest and bought myself some Rosary Beads to pray with.

At another point, I downloaded a Buddhist 'chanting' audio which I listened to daily for a while, contacted an online psychic lady who cast bespoke (and expensive) spells. I even toyed with the idea of running away from everything and everyone and joining a Convent to get away from alcohol. I bought Chinese herbal medicines and read books, online advice forums and inspirational quotes from sober celebrities who had conquered alcoholism - basically anything that I thought would help me to control or give up drinking.

Looking back it is almost heart-breaking to remember the vain attempts that I made to stop alcohol from ruining my life and the money that I wasted, and I know that I was in no way unique in this.

There are countless people like me going through this every day. I was constantly in search of a 'cure' and I wanted my life back so badly that I would believe in anyone who said that they could help me, but in between weird treatments, AA and rehab I would inevitably lapse and eventually pick up a drink again, forgetting how bad it had been. I would then begin the journey down the boring, destructive spiral all over again, each time becoming increasingly desperate.

Chapter 5

Rehab

This chapter has proved to be more challenging for me to write than I initially thought it would be, and I think that is because I know that rehab isn't even an option for most alcoholics, mainly due to the huge costs involved in staying there, so I know I was very fortunate in that respect. I also want to begin this chapter by stressing that on the two occasions I entered rehab, I was one hundred percent determined to do everything I was told and to make it work in order to get sober and stay that way.

This is because prior to entering rehab on both occasions, I was in a very bad way and had caused everyone around me major upset and worry. I was desperate to stop drinking. My stints in rehab may have been years apart and the outward signs of the severity of my alcoholism different, but the fundamental reason for me being there was the same - to be 'cured' of my alcoholism, and I wanted it to work so badly.

Because I attended rehab at different stages down the alcoholic spiral, and because the two facilities I attended couldn't have been more different in terms of their approach, their philosophy and their attitude towards their clients, I believe my experiences might help shed some light on why rehab is not the appropriate treatment for everyone. I know too well that awful, sick feeling of guilt and shame that an alcoholic feels when a kind friend or family member has paid for an expensive stint in rehab, but they start drinking again at some point after leaving. I became overwhelmed by cravings which I just couldn't fight anymore. I convinced myself that I wasn't as bad as some of the people I met in rehab and believed again that I could control my drinking, and would no longer drink in an alcoholic way.

There is no guarantee that checking into a rehab facility will help an alcoholic to achieve actual long term or life-long sobriety. I don't deny that I did benefit from my time in both facilities in certain ways, such as the things I learned about myself and my alcoholism, and I also met some genuinely lovely people there who desperately wanted to achieve sobriety and live a normal life - something that we all had in common. I also believe that, in the main, the people running and working in rehabs do have a desire to help clients and that this comes from a good place but, ultimately, I did pick up a drink again after leaving both facilities and so my time there cannot be considered to be an unmitigated success.

The shame and guilt that an alcoholic feels when they pick up a drink or 'fall off the wagon' after rehab is immense and this is compounded by the widely accepted belief that if rehab doesn't work the blame lies solely with the alcoholic, who didn't try hard enough or just didn't want to stay sober, (the same belief applies to AA). This belief is never challenged - consider the stories in the media about celebrities who are in and out of rehab facilities - it is never the rehab facility that is criticised or even questioned, but always the famous patient who has failed, and I have been guilty in the past, (before my own experiences in rehab), of assuming the same.

To me this is very convenient for those running rehabs because it ensures they are never held to account, and it's quite alarming how little actual evidence there is that rehab actually works, long term. Controlled studies are difficult to find and if rehabs do talk about their success rates they are, in my experience, referring to those people who complete their programme and not about alcoholics who achieve long term or life-long sobriety.

Because of this lack of accountability there is, sadly, the opportunity for people to take advantage of desperate alcoholics and their families, in the same way that some of the hypnotherapists that I saw took my money, even though they were not equipped to help me. There also seems to be a misguided perception that the more expensive a rehab is, the more expertise its staff must have and the more successful it must be, i.e. you get what you pay for.

I despair when I read about public figures entering rehab and allegedly nipping home or texting people and updating their social media, when the whole point is supposed to be to remove the alcoholic from outside influences and potential triggers and allow them to focus entirely on their recovery. It's easy to get the impression that the more it costs, the more clients are pandered to, which does not make any sense.

Being in rehab does, however, provide an opportunity to detox and I think that this is the very real benefit of being confined in a place that is geared up for caring for people who are stopping drinking, because detoxing is something that can be incredibly challenging to achieve at home. When you are in rehab you are, hopefully, completely removed from any opportunities to buy or obtain alcohol and any withdrawal symptoms are usually carefully monitored and managed from a medical perspective. The withdrawal that a chronic alcoholic experiences when they stop drinking can be absolutely horrific and very frightening, and alcohol is one drug which can actually cause death if you suddenly stop taking it.

Once you have detoxed in rehab, you will have several more weeks or even months when you don't have any access to alcohol, which allows your body to begin to recover and should enable you to 'rehabilitate' and explore your reasons for drinking and ways of coping with life without a drink.

In theory, an alcoholic should leave rehab completely detoxed and, more importantly, fully equipped with all of the mental tools necessary to lead a sober life and to be able to manage cravings, triggers and moments of weakness, and they should also have dealt with the underlying issues which lead to them becoming an alcoholic in the first place.

Sadly, this was not my experience, and although I left rehab full of hope and absolute resolve never to drink again, I was eventually beaten and worn down again by alcohol. Based on my own experience, I regard rehab as a very expensive way of keeping the alcoholic away from alcohol, an enforced period of abstinence, and I think that the long term success metrics of rehab facilities are not challenged enough.

I believe that this could be because alcoholics or their loved ones are in such an absolutely desperate place when they pick up the phone to a rehab facility, thoughts of asking for evidence of success are not foremost in their mind.

My own experiences with rehab began exactly like that, with an emotional phone call because I realised that I badly needed help when my drinking was out of control.

The first time I picked up the phone to a rehab I was racked with worry after my ex-husband and sister had been forced to break into my house, only to find me unconscious after drinking vodka. This was highly unusual for me then, and it would be quite a few years before my second stint in rehab or when I reached my own rock bottom, but way back then I was concerned enough about the impact alcohol was having on my life to search for somewhere that could hopefully help me.

The place I found that first time is, to me, a perfect example of how anyone, perhaps with the best of intentions, can set up a rehab facility, apparently without having a clue about what they're doing. It also demonstrates how my alcoholic head made me impulsive in my frantic search, and that I didn't do any real research about different places in order to make an informed choice.

I arrived there full of confidence and hope that I would leave sober and never drink again, and the staff were indisputably caring and friendly. It was in a beautiful remote country house a few hours drive from my home, and I was sober when I arrived. The facility had only very recently opened, which I hadn't realised when I booked it, and I was one of five people there, which under normal circumstances would be a real bonus in terms of individual attention, (my second rehab at times seemed to have too many clients at one time).

The emphasis was very much focused on a spiritual approach to tackling alcoholism, (the second rehab took a more traditional Twelve Step approach). However what at first appeared to be a relaxed and informal atmosphere quickly became a cause for concern for me when I realised that this approach was not deliberate, but had more to do with the fact that the facility was ineptly managed and very lax.

Out of the five clients, two really didn't want to be there and they were very honest about this. One was there as an alternative to going to prison, and the other to prevent their child being taken into care, but we all had the same goal of beating alcoholism, even if the reasons motivating us were different.

It became apparent to me that the people running the place and their underlying philosophies were 'alternative' to say the least and they seemed to dabble in a mish mash of ideas, without any real structure or overall plan, and for a lot of the time the five of us really didn't have a clue what was going on. We actually found this funny, which wasn't very helpful because we quickly developed a group 'naughty children' mentality rather than questioning whether any of what we were doing was helping us.

My daily routine always started with time spent sitting in front of a light box or 'phototherapy', which was meant to help with mood. While one person sat in front of the light box, the others just chatted and had coffee, and the mood very quickly became jovial, not at all what I had imagined rehab would be like.

The treatments that we took part in ranged from swinging crystals over us as we lay on the floor, to a trip to a local supermarket to walk down the alcohol aisle in order to explore how it felt. I once had a very strange one to one chat with the owner of the facility, when he told me about Native American approaches to addiction, and the sweat lodge that he was planning to build in the grounds.

An elderly nurse was supposed to be on duty in the house every night, with the owner and other staff leaving at five o clock daily. Unbelievably, after about a week into my stay there, the nurse said she was unable to stay overnight for health reasons. The owner gave me the keys because I was considered to be the most sensible and left the five of us 'inmates' on our own.

I was the only one there who had arrived in a car, and after about ten weird and wonderful days, I was persuaded to drive to the local supermarket one evening when we had been left on our own and we bought alcohol and took it back to the house. I am ashamed of this even now, but at the time the whole situation had turned into a surreal joke and we found every day hilarious - it was like being in a strange boarding school with a bunch of naughty kids.

It's hard to believe that less than two weeks before this I had been sitting in front of the GP with my sisters, crying and begging for help and here I was drunk and laughing at my situation, and convincing myself that the vodka incident had been a one off.

I was remorseful enough after the alcohol incident to do what was the decent thing in my eyes, and cut my stay at the rehab short mainly because I felt so guilty for enabling my new friends to potentially jeopardise their future by breaking the rules underpinning their stay in rehab.

I returned home and convinced everyone that I was rehabilitated and able to drink in a 'normal' way, and that the events leading up to my stay in rehab had been out of the ordinary. This was nine years before my 'rock bottom', and I acknowledge that I wasn't ready to even contemplate giving up alcohol forever back then.

Despite the strange set up of this first rehab, there were a couple of positive elements that I took away with me, that have become more important to me since I got sober.

The most important was my introduction to Dr Joe Dispenza, who appeared in a film that we were shown one afternoon called 'What The Bleep Do We Know'. At the time the film seemed way above my head because much of the content focuses on the field of quantum physics, which I had absolutely no knowledge of. However, Dr Joe Dispenza talked briefly in the film about 'creating your day', which somehow stayed with me and I later discovered that he was really explaining the science behind the book The Secret, which my son Michael bought for me several years later. It wouldn't be until years later when I remembered the video and bought some of Dr Joe Dispenza's books that I realised this, and I talk about this more in Chapter 10.

The other positive aspect from my time in that first rehab which has stayed with me, was a recording of myself stating affirmations, which had been placed over a soundtrack that they had created from the rhythms of my own body, (they did this by putting a monitor on my finger which picked up my heartbeat and breathing). Again, very weird and completely beyond the realms of my own understanding and experience, but it sounds quite haunting and beautiful and I have kept a copy of it to this very day. I believe that this rehab centre closed after just a couple of years.

The second rehab that I attended was the complete opposite of the first, and the circumstances which lead me there several years down the line were far more serious. My alcoholism had by then reached crisis point and my husband Ross had been forced to reach out to Mark's Mum for help after I had been hospitalised and the police had been involved in our lives because of my drinking.

This rehab was much more traditional in approach, and I was required to hand over my mobile phone and bank cards on entering. I wasn't allowed any contact with my family for what seemed like an age, but I was happy to do this because I was in such a hopeless state by then and crying out again for help.

The second rehab came highly recommended by word of mouth, and I learned that some of the people who were there at the same time as me had previously attended other more well-known addiction centres, only to sadly relapse and go in search for an alternative. I felt wretched when I walked through the doors because my being there had forced Ross to cancel our family holiday, and I would also miss Michael's eighteenth birthday, but my family didn't care about those things, they just wanted me to get sober and to be the Mum and wife that they loved again. I was so sad and frightened, but I believed one hundred percent that this would be the place that would save me. I also knew that I was incredibly lucky because the rehab was incredibly expensive and had been paid for by Mark's Mum, which was so very loving and kind, and more than I felt I deserved

The rehabilitation was based around the Twelve Step approach, as well as group therapy and one to one counselling, and we lived under very strict conditions without mobile phones or the internet and only limited and supervised trips outside. This filled me with confidence because, unlike my first rehab, everything was highly organised and structured and the staff there were very professional. I surrendered myself to the process there and put my faith in them completely. After years of my alcohol progressing and then the alarming rate that it had escalated recently, I knew that I had reached the stage where, if I didn't beat it, I was going to lose everything.

And so I began my time there as I meant to go on. I wanted to get as much as possible out of my stay and I needed to return home sober with the ability to avoid the temptation to drink again. In one of my first sessions there I was asked to write down words that I would use to describe myself and I wrote 'bad mother, selfish, unreliable, pathetic and self-destructive' and that was genuinely how I felt.

I was ashamed of myself and scared of the future, but I was glad that any feelings of self-pity were immediately squashed. For example, in one interactive session when I put my hand up to say that I wanted to beat alcoholism because Michael was my life, I was scoffed at by the counsellor who said, 'yeah, he's so much your life that you've spent years getting pissed and not giving him a second thought'. I liked this tough approach and knew that it was true.

I also found learning about the reasons behind addiction fascinating and helpful, and I met some fantastic people there, including some of the staff. They even invited Ross in for a family session, and encouraged Ross, Michael and anyone else close to me to write letters explaining the impact that my drinking had on them. This was incredibly humbling and a wake-up call. People are often frightened to be honest with alcoholics, and the stress that this puts on families is unfair. This was an opportunity for them to tell me honestly how damaging my behaviour was and how it made them feel. I am truly grateful that they were given the opportunity to do that in a way that would not make them feel any guilt or worry about how I would react.

While I was glad that my self-pity and ego were swiftly squashed upon entering this rehab, sadly I found much of my time there very challenging for the wrong reasons, with the group therapy and one to one counselling creating more problems for me than they actually solved.

I'm sure that group therapy can be incredibly useful in certain situations, but I found it completely detrimental and even observed at times that it had a damaging impact on some of the people that I was with. Like I said, it was only right that everyone was made to feel 'equal' and the removal of ego and being humble and vulnerable was a useful thing, because alcoholics can be very self-absorbed. However I believe that the group therapy could sometimes do more harm than good for a number of reasons.

Just as with AA groups, rehab throws together a mixed bag of people, where the common denominator is the desire to stop drinking and to stop destroying their lives and those of their families. However, as with any random group of people, you get all of the different personality types - show offs, attention seekers, bullies, cool people, teachers pets, shy people, disruptive people, lecherous people.... etc.

This can prove problematic in a group therapy situation because often the same few people will tend to dominate the situation, whether that's because they want to talk about themselves or to be generally disruptive.

I found myself becoming increasingly frustrated until one day, about one week into my time there I stood up and said, "I have been here for one week and not once have I been asked to share my story in this group. You know nothing about me, but we all know everything about a few people here".

I don't think that the situation there was helped by the fact that people entered and left the rehab in a fluid way, so some of the people in the group had been there for weeks or months and were very obviously bored.

The staff facilitating the group therapy sometimes seemed almost star struck by some of the 'cool' people there, and there was also a very uncomfortable and subtle 'bullying' culture of one man in particular, simply because he was slightly nerdy.

There is a fine line between the tough love that I mentioned earlier and bullying, and one staff member in particular seemed to get pleasure out of singling him out in group therapy and making him feel embarrassed. I felt so sorry for him and am ashamed that I didn't try to stand up for him.

The potential harm of group therapy for me was also highlighted by the fact that people become alcoholics for so many different reasons, so you might have someone in a room that has been sexually abused as a child and someone who is creepy and lecherous and doesn't understand physical boundaries.

I can remember pouring out my heart in one session, and an often disruptive older woman just bursting out laughing and mocking me – I felt crushed and embarrassed. The fact that there is no escape from each other either, because you are there 24 / 7 for weeks or months, can create further tension.

One of the reasons that the group therapy was so challenging, I believe, was the fact that there were just far too many people in the room at one time. I am in no doubt that this is about maximising profit, rather than a desire to help everyone, and I am sure that the second rehab I attended will not be the only facility guilty of this.

The fact that there were so many people there also impacted on the one to one sessions that we were promised. Because of the client to staff ratio, I found that in the five weeks that I was there, I only had three one to one counselling sessions with two different people.

The very real and potentially harmful danger of this, is that it just scratches the surface of any underlying problems or brings to light something that has been buried deep inside for years. There is then the real risk that, because something has been uncovered and not dealt with, real emotional harm may be done to the person. Again, I am sure that this will not be unique to the rehab that I attended, but I found my sporadic counselling sessions detrimental to my emotional wellbeing.

I can remember that several times we were all reminded, by different members of staff, that statistically only two or three out of every ten of us would achieve sobriety, and that the rest would never beat alcoholism and it would kill them. I have heard and read these statistics many times over the years, but to be reminded of that in rehab seemed almost like a 'get out of jail card' for them.

Can you imagine that sort of statement being accepted with a defeatist shrug in any other medical treatment? I can't, and I found it really frightening and confusing when we were given this warning. Even if it was intended to help us by scaring us into trying harder so that we didn't become a sad statistic, it seemed like an excuse for failure. Were they implying that the majority of us who were there simply didn't want sobriety enough? I wanted it desperately.

Like I said, I don't think that the second rehab that I attended was out of the ordinary; in fact it had a very good reputation. I just feel frustrated that the whole rehab industry has been unaccountable for years and there aren't enough real statistics about long term success rates for desperate people to make an informed decision. Rehab costs an absolute fortune and is not available to the majority of alcoholics, and the only knowledge most people have about rehab is when they see a story about rock star excess on the front of a tabloid newspaper or they watch a guest on the Jeremy Kyle show being sent to a facility.

I know that some will consider me to be ungrateful or say that I failed because I didn't try, because that is how it goes for every alcoholic who spends time being 'rehabilitated' and then picks up a drink again. It is their fault alone. While I was there I reminded myself constantly about how lucky I was, and that I was only there because I had so much love around me - even then. I also kept telling myself that it must work because so many people go into rehab, and so I had to squash any feelings of doubt or discomfort in group therapy - we were doing it for a reason.

And so, when I left the second rehab after five weeks, I was absolutely determined that I was never going to pick up a drink again. I did everything that I was told including going to meetings, and I felt genuinely excited for the future. As I describe in Chapter 3, I did feel like a duck out of water and paranoid that everyone was watching me, but I worked incredibly hard to simply not pick up that first drink.

But that is the problem, it still came down to my own willpower and self-control, and the pull of alcohol was so strong that it eventually became too overwhelming. I again convinced myself that I would be able to control my drinking because I needed a drink so much and also, (the same old story), I told myself that I was not as bad as some of the people that I had met in rehab.

I did call to talk to someone there and told them that I was struggling and I was told that I wasn't going to enough AA meetings, which was probably true.

In retrospect, maybe I should have gone to a rehab which was closer to home, which was easier to maintain connections with for support after I left.

I feel that ultimately, I was simply kept away from alcohol for five weeks, but the dark shadow was still there in the background, waiting for the right time to whisper to me again. This is the reality of alcoholism, it robs you of all of your loyalties and your moral compass and I believed again that if I could hide it from everyone that everything would be okay - I just had to have a drink.

And so I know the shame and guilt that comes with picking up a drink after someone has spent a fortune on rehab fees. After the people who loved me most had made sacrifices for me to be there, all the while showing me nothing but love and support. My husband had attended a family meeting there and poured his heart out, and my son Michael was so happy to have me home and sober. And, because I believed that this was one hundred percent my failure, because rehab should have worked for me, the feelings of self-loathing and self-hatred were immense. The dark shadow took charge and sidled up to me once more.

Very soon my alcoholism was worse than it had been before I had entered rehab.

Chapter 6

AA

I think it's safe to say that the majority of alcoholics will have some experience of AA. When you're absolutely desperate and don't know where to turn, someone will always answer the phone when you dial the AA telephone number, and I think that simple act and the almost guaranteed warmth and compassion that greets someone who has found themselves in the depths of despair with alcohol, has almost certainly saved many people.

In that moment, when you reach out because you're drunk or hungover, or have found yourself in a position where everyone around you is at the end of their patience, and you're frightened and alone, AA is often the only place left to turn.

I've found myself dialling the AA number many times over the years, but the most significant time was when I started drinking again after a few months of sobriety, following my second stay in rehab. It was incredible how quickly I found myself in exactly the same dark place (mentally and physically) as I had been just before I went into rehab, and with my relationships with Ross and Michael at crisis point. I was staying at my friend Vicky's house at the time, because Ross had to go away on business the day after he had found me at home horribly drunk a few months after I left residential treatment. He had reached the end of his tether and Michael had left home disgusted and upset with me.

I attended an AA meeting near to where Vicky lived, but after I moved back home when Ross returned from his business trip, I promised him that I would follow a strict timetable of AA meetings in our area. Ross had heard it all before, but I was determined that I would do it properly - everything now depended on it, and I was desperate for help - I cannot adequately describe the sick feeling you have when you know that you'll lose absolutely everything if you let people down again.

When you've failed at rehab and all attempts at keeping yourself sober, giving AA one hundred percent commitment seems all there is left, and I'm forever grateful that they were there at that time in my life.

The lady who answered my call could not have been more caring and reassuring. She was kindness itself and arranged to meet me and take me to a meeting very close to our home, (she eventually became my Sponsor). Turning up at an AA meeting alone can be quite daunting, even when the people are friendly and welcoming, (which they are in the majority of cases), and being introduced to people and included in conversations in the break filled me with a warm sense of belonging and immense hope that these people could help me to live an alcohol free life.

I was upset and broken, cutting quite a pathetic figure, but I was accepted with open arms, and that to me is the uniquely special thing about AA – the many wonderful individuals that you find at meetings, who understand exactly what you are going through and what you are putting your loved ones through.

I immediately liked the people that I met that night, and it was to become my 'home' group, the group that I wanted to be part of, and the weekly meeting that I didn't want to miss.

Around these 'home' meetings, I timetabled in meetings slightly further afield to fill my week, so that I never went more than a couple of days without a meeting in my diary. This included a meeting for women only, where women can discuss things that they may feel uncomfortable discussing in front of men. Because AA groups are organised and run by the members themselves with, (hopefully), no 'hierarchy' or leaders, there are different kinds of meetings that have evolved over time. Some of the groups I attended would have one person 'share' their story and in others we would go around the room and take turns talking about how our week had been.

Since AA is all about anonymity and, in their view, I should not even be talking about the fact that I have been to meetings, out of respect for the people I met through AA, I will not go into specifics about the meetings that I attended over the following months. I do, however, need to talk in general about my experiences, good and bad because, just like rehab, the fact that attending regular AA meetings did not keep me sober is one of my main reasons for writing this book. This is to reassure others experiencing the same problems that I did that they are not alone, and also to give their frustrated loved ones a better understanding of why AA might not work.

The lady who I first talked to on the telephone was a beautiful soul and immediately took me under her wing and made me feel safe. She became my friend as well as my Sponsor. AA is full of truly kind people who want to help fellow alcoholics and who want to stay sober themselves, which can make it an incredibly powerful source of support and encouragement. People look out for each other and notice if someone is struggling or hasn't turned up to meetings for a while, and because the only requirement for being part of AA is a desire to stop drinking, there is always a welcome, even if you turn up drunk or have started to drink again in between meetings.

Over the following few months I very enthusiastically got involved with the various groups I attended, which was made easier for me because, undeservedly, I still had my driving license and could attend lots of different meetings. I asked the lady who had taken me under her wing to be my Sponsor and I began to work the Twelve Steps of AA with her guidance, something that I had not attempted before. We would meet regularly outside of meetings and I enjoyed not just the fact that I was doing things properly this time, but also the fact that she was so wise and seemed to understand me. Our friendship became very important to me.

When the time came for me to do the Third Step and turn my life over to a Higher Power, (because I had accepted in Step 1 that I was powerless over alcohol), we went to Durham Cathedral to do this, which I found overwhelmingly powerful and emotional. I felt full of hope and strength for the first time in ages and I believed that this time I was really going to beat my alcoholism.

AA is by no means a religious organisation, however I understand that many people struggle with the 'Higher Power' element because it seems to allude to 'God', but I never felt like that. I was just happy to believe that something more powerful than me, even some hidden strength inside me, was going to keep me sober - because I needed to believe it.

I had tried and failed to stay sober so many times that if you had told me to put my hand in a fire and I would never drink alcohol again, I would've gladly done it. I also completely signed up to Step 1, accepting that I was completely powerless over alcohol.

Again, many critics of AA have difficulty with this concept because it suggests that you have no free will, and some see it as an attempt to relinquish blame. To be honest, I really don't care about an in depth analysis of the Steps or of the psychology behind my alcoholism, I just knew then, as I still know about myself now, that if I ever had a drink I would want to continue to drink until I was completely drunk or pass out, and so I regarded myself as powerless over it, which made putting my faith in the Steps easy for me - at that moment in time.

As the weeks passed and Ross and Michael could see that I was attending regular meetings and committing myself fully to AA, things at home did begin to slowly improve. I didn't expect Michael to move back home completely and I certainly didn't deserve that, but he did begin to spend more time with us, and they were both very encouraging and interested in hearing about my meetings and what I did with my Sponsor.

I engrossed myself in AA literature, including the Big Book, and I felt a massive sense of relief that I had finally reached that point in my life where I was strong enough to resist alcohol, manage any cravings and rebuild my life and relationships - getting the real me back. Seeing people come and go within AA, starting to drink again, dying or just simply disappearing never to be heard of again, was always very sad, and a powerful warning that our dark shadow is always there waiting, alcohol in hand. I still believe that to this day, but observing first-hand how seemingly strong people who had been sober for years could just suddenly 'fall off the wagon' was absolutely heart wrenching and a very powerful lesson - alcohol never, ever gives up on trying to tempt you back.

Within the rooms of AA meetings, I listened intently to other people's stories when they 'shared' and I gladly shared mine too. There was always some element of every story that we could all relate to and remind ourselves of how bad things had been, and how hideous our lives would become if we ever picked up a drink again.

But this is where the AA experience for me began to become problematic. I began to feel like I would never move forward if I was constantly having to remind myself of what an awful person I had been, and recounting all of the damage I had done to everyone who cared about me over and over for the rest of my life.

Now at this point I understand that many would accuse me of looking for excuses while I was attending AA to ensure that it failed, deliberately fixating on the negative in order to justify the fact that I eventually started drinking again. This is not true and I can say this emphatically because I know how much I wanted AA to work for me with every fibre of my body – I needed it to work because my life depended on it, as well as my relationships with Michael and Ross.

AA has been the 'gold standard' treatment for alcoholics for years, and questioning anything about AA within a meeting or with your sponsor would be regarded as 'impolite' at best, stirring up trouble or, the old faithful, a sign that you're still in denial.

Because I felt 'ungrateful' for feeling like this and having uncertainty, and because I was obviously worried that it was my dark shadow whispering to my alcoholic head and trying to confuse me and tempt me away from AA, I tried to squash any niggling doubts and to just focus on making it work.

But the thought of reinforcing the negative and regurgitating all of the truly horrible and shameful things that I had done whilst drunk, on a regular basis for the rest of my life, began to really bother me. I will never forget and would not want to forget, how bad things became and what a dark place I have been in many times during my life, but I do not think that it is healthy or even effective as a method of maintaining sobriety to pour over things again and again, or even to listen to the harrowing 'shares' of others week in week out.

By constantly reminding myself of my embarrassing, destructive, dangerous and even illegal behaviour, as well as the hurt that I had caused to other people, I believe that I could never escape alcohol and 'move on' to create a completely alcohol free and positive life. But that is what I did and what many alcoholics all over the world do in order to stay sober and stay alive. This means facing the prospect of alcohol remaining a huge part of your life 24/7, for the rest of your life.

So even if I wasn't drinking, I would be battling thoughts about drinking and reliving and recounting my alcoholic horror stories from time to time and listening to the stories of others several times a week. I would never be able to completely 'draw a line' underneath my alcoholism.

I can vividly imagine us all sitting there in the room, with our dark shadows hovering around us to listen to our stories and while we recounted the hideous things we had done whilst drunk, the hurt and the shame we felt, the dark shadows are congratulating each other on the chaos they had caused and feeling empowered. We were keeping them alive and feeding them by talking like this, when I just wanted to escape mine forever.

Inevitably, because I had this uneasy feeling about this aspect of AA, meetings for me started to become quite negative experiences. In my understanding, the only way to maintain sobriety was to attend regular meetings for the rest of my life, reminding myself ad nauseam of the dark places that alcohol had taken me to.

I remember a woman of around fifteen years sobriety telling me that she couldn't ever allow alcohol in the house and felt uncomfortable around people who were drinking because she could feel 'that old feeling' stirring, her dark shadow never far from her side, now pricking up its ears. I imagined myself hanging onto sobriety by my fingertips day in, day out forever, alcohol and my dark shadow always there in the background trying to wear me down.

I now strongly believe that dwelling on the negative events of the past and constantly declaring to everyone that you're an alcoholic does feed alcoholism with 'energy', keeping it alive and well and a part of your life forever. Even the act of saying, 'Hi, I'm Sue and I'm an alcoholic' every time I wanted to speak never allowed me to move on from that, as if it was now my defining feature. I understand that the reason for doing this is to maintain 'humility' because it's important that everyone at AA is seen as being equal, but wouldn't it be far more positive and empowering to say, 'Hi, I'm Sue and I'm a recovering alcoholic', or 'I'm not drinking today'?

The fact is that AA is a lifelong commitment and they believe without question (and it is always made very clear), that if you do not regularly attend AA meetings you will relapse, and if someone did relapse or just stopped coming to meetings, it was always because they hadn't worked the programme properly.

There is a widespread belief that the only proven way for alcoholics to beat their addiction is to attend AA meetings until they die and to be reminded of how bad life was when they were drinking. Many rehabs, including the second one I was treated in, advise that clients follow a Twelve Step programme once they leave their care. I was brought up as a Catholic and went to Catholic school, and it reminds me of the way the fear of hell was used to frighten us into being 'good' children.

But this was not the only reason why I think that AA didn't work for me. As with any institution that we might become part of throughout our lives including school and the workplace, (and rehab), AA was a mixed bag of people from all walks of life with every kind of personality type. The fact that we all had alcoholism in common did not mean that everyone was kind, caring and supportive, (although the majority of people I met were). You still found the leaders, the gossips, the mean people, the weirdos, the lechers, the bullies – they were all there and sometimes this could make the experience of attending meetings uncomfortable or even disturbing.

In some meetings there were impenetrable 'cliques' who didn't welcome new people, and in others there were overly familiar people who wanted to get to know you a little too enthusiastically. This is true in every aspect of life. It's part of human nature and doesn't present your average adult with any problems, but when you're struggling with something like alcoholism, you really don't need another layer of anxiety in your life, and I sometimes found it difficult to deal with. I can remember trying hard to become part of some AA groups, especially with some of the women, and finding it very difficult. I would often find myself changing my behaviour, for example smoking more than I should or joining in with gossip, in order to be accepted.

Someone once said to me during a meeting that some AA meetings are a 'hotbed of mental health issues' - I certainly had my own issues - and when you put all of these people together at varying stages of their struggle with alcohol, it can be challenging. In my eagerness to feel accepted and ingratiate myself with the various AA groups, I willingly offered lifts to people, picking them up and dropping them off after meetings, because this was one way that I knew that I could be useful.

Being so eager to please lead to one very uncomfortable situation when one woman that I became friendly with declared to the whole group that she was in love with me, and told me privately that she wanted to take things further. After that I felt I could no longer attend the meetings that she went to, I just couldn't handle having to deal with unwanted romantic attention on top of trying to stay sober.

It probably seems trivial, reading it on a page, but you have to put situations like this into context. I was battling an addiction, trying to make amends and to win back the trust and respect of my family, (and hopefully, eventually, get back some self-respect and self-esteem), whilst trying to negotiate the internal politics of the AA groups, and the sometimes startling behaviour of the people within them.

Although the majority of people you meet at meetings really want to be there and are very motivated, some people you come across aren't there of their own free will, because it can sometimes be a requirement of the courts that people follow a Twelve Step programme in order to regain custody of their children or stay out of prison (for example).

Sometimes there are people there who want to prey on new vulnerable members, befriending them with less than caring intentions. Anyone who has spent a reasonable amount of time in AA, (or rehab), becomes aware of the Thirteenth Step, when someone who has been around AA for a while tries to have sex with a vulnerable newcomer by gaining their trust through being caring and helpful and showing them lots of attention. As I said before, I myself tried very hard to be 'liked' and to fit in, so it is easy to see how this eagerness and naivety could potentially be exploited by some men and women.

Because I knew that this was my last chance to get sober, and since I had tried and failed with everything else, I told myself that all of these doubts and niggling worries I had about AA were, in fact, alcohol and my dark shadow trying to pull me away from my meetings and my Sponsor. Alcohol never gives up trying to draw you back into having that first drink, and so I continued with my meetings and the Twelve Steps, attending the annual, one day, regional AA Convention and generally trying very hard not to drink.

There were also many positive things about being part of AA which I clung on to, and I absolutely loved the genuinely caring people that I met, especially my Sponsor, and the support that those people give each other is very moving and honest. The amazing feeling that you get when everyone holds hands at the end of a meeting to say the Serenity Prayer is so powerful and fills you with such hope that I always left the room feeling very optimistic. The Serenity Prayer is still important to me today because I think it applies to everyone, regardless of their relationship to addiction.

I do understand that the feeling of being part of something, having the community of support and friendship and even just the regular company of people, is a real benefit to many, and I don't wish to take that away from AA. There is also a lot of wisdom in many of the AA philosophies, especially keeping it simple, which was something that I only really grasped much later down the line in my alcoholic journey.

The fact that they also stress that you should only try to make amends with people if you won't cause that person more hurt or harm by doing so, is also important and wise advice. I have not tried to build bridges with some of the people that I hurt when I was drunk, even now, because I know that it would mainly be for my own benefit, to make myself feel better. I now believe that those people are better off living their lives without me contacting them or dragging up the past again.

However, as I detail in Chapter 3, attending AA and throwing myself into working the Twelve Steps ultimately didn't work for me, and I eventually did have that first drink. I know that this is down to my own complete lack of willpower around alcohol, but I want to refer back to the heart breaking notes that I wrote to Michael and Ross which I shared at the end of Chapter 3, and tell you how inconceivable and how tragic it is to me now that I could've felt so bereft and sorry, and to be absolutely pleading for forgiveness, and then a few months down the line start drinking again. I needed to make AA work and I did try very hard.

I know that AA stalwarts will say that I didn't work the programme properly and that anyone who does will not pick up a drink it even says so in 'The Big Book', which AA members are guided by –

"...those who do not recover are those who cannot or will not give themselves completely to this simple program, usually men and women who are constitutionally incapable of being honest with themselves. There are such unfortunates..."

But I knew that this was my last chance and I knew that if it didn't work I would lose everything, and that probably included my life, and I did give myself to their programme - but still alcohol won again. I began to compare myself to other people in AA, people who had lost their children to social services, or lost their job and I felt that I wasn't as big an alcoholic as they were. Absolutely insane and amnesic logic because Michael was older by now and had moved out several times to live with his Dad, and I didn't have a job to lose – but if I did, I would've been sacked a very long time ago.

I allowed the whole 'forever' thing to fill me with panic. I didn't want maintaining sobriety to mean having to fit my whole life around meetings forever – I didn't want my sobriety to impact on our home life forever. This seems crazy because at that time the only alternative was being an active alcoholic, which massively and negatively impacted on our lives. Maybe I just wasn't suited to AA, maybe I wasn't ready or lacked the willpower of people who make it work.

Whatever the reason, my behaviour again became destructive and unforgivable. I began to secretly drink on my way home after meetings. Soon I found myself pretending to go to meetings, but instead I would sit in a car park somewhere drinking. This made me feel wretched with guilt for letting down Michael, Ross and my Sponsor, but I also started to grow afraid that I was crossing over a line the point of no return. I absolutely hated myself. My life became even more of a lie than it had ever been, and nothing seemed real anymore.

I know that I am far from unique and that AA does not work for many people. It is actually very difficult to find any concrete statistics around the success rate of AA. Some have claimed that the figure is as low as five percent, but statistics aren't important when you just want to be in the successful group. I certainly saw many people come and go and, I now know that some people that I met there have since died because of their alcoholism. This is tragic, because the majority of people who find themselves in the rooms of AA fiercely want to stop drinking and get their lives back.

What is frustrating for me is that AA as an organisation could make such a huge difference if their philosophy didn't seem so 'closed', because they have an audience of people at every meeting who could benefit so much from hearing different kinds of success stories. For example, I believe that I would not be welcome at an AA meeting now to talk about how I won back my sobriety and my life, because I don't attribute my success to AA.

Surely the ultimate goal should be to help people get sober by sharing positive stories. There should be an openness, and a desire to listen to anyone who has conquered their own alcoholism, in the same way that the medical profession share examples of 'best practice' with each other.

'To heal a wound you have to stop touching it', or so goes the saying, but at AA you are touching it over and over again, so that it never heals. On top of that, it seems to me that you're repeatedly reinforcing the negative, giving your alcoholism energy by talking about it constantly, and listening to stories about the chaos it has caused, week in week out.

No matter how many months or years of sobriety you rack up, if you pick up a drink, all of your previous achievements are erased and you start counting your sobriety again from Day 1. You can never say 'forever', but have to work at it one day at a time, which I found all-consuming and draining. It's a battle that many people lose, including me.

And so, when I picked up a drink after all my hard work in AA, and began to lie to everyone again, I felt completely defeated and broken, and now there was nothing else left that could help me.

Chapter 7

Rock Bottom

Being in the grip of active alcoholism is the most terrifying and desperately lonely place I have ever been, but nothing prepared me for how much worse things became, and the despair and sense of foreboding which consumed me at the beginning of 2015.

The way in which my alcoholism had escalated so quickly over the previous eighteen months was alarming. I progressed from being what I might have called an 'average' alcoholic, who goes to meetings and counselling, spends time in rehab, sobers up, falls of the wagon, gets back on the wagon and so on to being unable to stop drinking.

Where once there was naïve optimism that I had a chance of becoming a 'normal' drinker again, I was now starting to realise with a horrible, fatalistic certainty, that I could never beat it, and there were no more options available to me. It was heart breaking.

I was completely defeated by alcohol and felt that I couldn't live without it, and the creeping realisation that I was going to die sooner rather than later was overwhelmingly terrifying. I still tear up just remembering the sense of total despair that I felt, and the realisation that any efforts to be 'normal' again were futile.

It hadn't escaped me that you don't tend to see very old 'active' alcoholics, (unless someone has become an alcoholic in later life) and here I was, destined to make my contribution to the alarming statistics for alcohol related deaths.

I had spent so many years denying that I had a problem with alcohol and then many more trying to fight and beat it. Two stints in rehab, years of AA meetings and various other 'treatments' including counselling, SMART therapy and five different hypnotherapists in different parts of the country, had all failed.

Now it had me exactly where alcohol wants an alcoholic, lost, alone and terrified, but unable to stop drinking. The dark shadow that had the sole purpose of harming me and destroying my life from the beginning had won and was now like a parasite, eating me from inside. A slow suicide.

A few months before my rock bottom, I was in a very dark and secret place. It had been a year since I left my last rehab and months since I had picked up a drink and had got horribly drunk waiting for Ross to come back from a work trip. This had ended in a nasty accident slicing potatoes with a mandolin and everyone quickly becoming aware that I had fallen off the wagon again, only a few months after a fortune had been spent on my stint in rehab. They were all very disappointed and, understandably, totally fed up with me.

The day after my accident, Ross had to leave me in the care of my friend Vicky, because he had to go away and during those few days staying at her house, I started going to AA meetings again. I felt completely wretched and remorseful, and I was determined to give AA everything I could - again.

Poor Michael was so angry with me he just couldn't forgive me and he went off to live at his Dad's – again. He was in his A Level year and I was doing a fantastic job of messing it up for him.

Yet again I had been full of remorse and yet again those close to me began to forgive me and try to get back to normality. After putting my heart and soul into working the twelve steps and attending meetings several times a week for months, I had, unbelievably to me now, found myself drinking after meetings, because I began to believe that I could now finally control my drinking and keep it a secret, even from my sponsor.

I convinced myself that I wasn't as far down the alcoholic spiral as many of the people that I met at AA. I told myself that it would be okay to drink to keep myself 'topped up', as long as I never got drunk, and as long as no one ever suspected. I also convinced myself that I would be able to do this forever and that everyone would be happy.

At this point I need to refer you back to the notes I wrote which I shared at the end of Chapter 3, to emphasise how appalled this makes me feel, and what an utter betrayal it was to Ross and Michael. They had trusted me because of the promises I had made when I started to drink again a few months after coming out of rehab, because I had begged and pleaded for forgiveness, and I had promised them that I would never drink again.

But now I was living a life full of lies again and the only time that this felt wrong, was when I tried to give up drinking for a few days. This would cause me to suffer from the all-consuming anxiety that an alcoholic experiences with withdrawal, when I would be overwhelmed by guilt and shame and a feeling of impending doom.

I had 'sensibly' decided to try to stick to drinking wine, after ending up in hospital the year before after downing vodka, and I convinced myself again that I could handle wine because it was the devil that I knew. However, as all alcoholics know, when you start drinking again after a period of sobriety, you soon surpass even the darkest times and worst moments that you experienced before, and the devastating consequences of your alcoholism intensify very quickly.

It didn't take long for my life to begin to unravel. I found that I couldn't even make a trip to the shops without buying a miniature of wine to have whilst I was out, as well as drinking after AA meetings and when I was alone at home. I was able to keep it a secret for a short time, and even managed to be a support for Ross when his Mum died suddenly in the summer, but I began to drink more and more, and both Michael and Ross began to suspect that I was drinking again, only this time, there were no big scenes, confrontations or frantic searches for my hidden stash of alcohol, simply because they had now switched off.

After the summer, Michael started a new chapter of his life at University and Ross started a new job three hundred miles away, which meant that he had to stay away from Monday to Friday. They had been through so much over recent years with my drinking and they knew that my promises from earlier in the year had now been broken, and I know it was a relief for them to be away from me and not to have to watch as I slowly destroyed myself. I was still lying to them about my drinking and my efforts to give up, trying to convince them that I was in control, but by then I could see that they knew I was lying.

I can still see the looks on their faces, a mixture of pity and contempt when they were faced with me, my eyes glazed, vehemently denying that I had been drinking. Over time, people living with an alcoholic adapt to the events that occur and situations that would alarm other people become normal and cease to shock.

They had both tried so hard over the years to help me, but I think they both felt they could do no more. It must be so difficult to watch someone you love killing themselves but, ultimately, life goes on for everyone around an alcoholic, and there comes a point when it's so draining and painful for families and friends that they give up. I have met many alcoholics who have lost everyone they love in their life, and it must be so heart-breaking for family members and friends to throw in the towel and walk away from someone who is drunk or unconscious all of the time. For them it must be like bereavement because they have, effectively, lost the person that they know and love. In a strange way, it was a relief that my husband and son were spared the pain and guilt of having to actually 'leave' me, and a fortunate coincidence for them that University and work meant that they didn't have to be around me.

The fact is, everyone has their own lives to lead, things move on for those around an alcoholic. They cannot be permanent babysitters, and so it was with us. With Michael and Ross removed from the situation because of circumstances, they could get some kind of normality back in their lives and be free of the chaos, pain and worry that comes with living with an alcoholic. I missed them both and the reality of Michael leaving home for good hit me very badly, but unlike most mothers, I used this to justify getting wasted when I was alone. I remember Michael sending me a picture of a little chilli plant that he had bought for his student room and I felt so ashamed that he still cared enough to do that.

And so I came up with a plan which I decided would help me to get alcoholism out of my system once and for all. Ross and I already had practical plans in terms of living arrangements. We would sell our house and I would eventually move south to be with him. Regardless of what happened, we decided we would have a final Christmas at our house in the north and I would move to be with him after that. So, in my mind, that gave me a few final months of drinking secretly during the week, and I vowed to give up completely when I moved to be with my husband permanently. I honestly believed that this freedom to drink whatever I wanted during the week would make it become boring, and then ultimately wouldn't feel the need to drink anymore. This must be unbelievable to any right-minded person - because it was obviously a deranged notion.

Alcoholics do this all of the time. In AA and rehab they call it 'doing a geographical', which basically means that you move away from familiar places, people and other 'triggers' and start afresh, in the belief that life will somehow be miraculously different when you're somewhere new, and your alcoholism will not follow you. It fills the alcoholic with hope and excitement, and I was no different. I genuinely believed that this was my opportunity to get alcohol out of my system by having no one to police me during the week, and my move south would then be a line in the sand and a completely fresh start.

For me, this meant that I was free to drink and sleep, drink and sleep, and not have to face Ross, Michael or anyone else. So, that was how I started to live. Drinking all week and trying to sober up for my husband coming back at weekends.

I would drink until I slept and maybe wake up at strange hours and drink some more. I would wake up and throw up and then start drinking again. This quickly became my normal, and it seemed okay to me. As long as nobody knew, as long as I dipped into my business and emails now and then, I believed that I wasn't doing any harm. It honestly felt like an ideal life to me and I rationalised this all to myself, as alcoholics do.

I loved Michael more than anything but I had totally messed up as a mother and now he had left home. All that was left was regret and emptiness, so I was drinking more than ever to blot this out - and the quantities rapidly increased. Because there were no time constraints on my days during the week anymore, I was effectively drinking over the whole 24 hours, interspersed with a couple of hours 'unconscious' here and there. To me, this new life made perfect sense. I thought that I could wallow in self-pity for a while, get it out of my system and then start a new, sober chapter in the south of England with Ross.

If I had to meet friends or family, who all believed at this point that I was on the wagon, I would try to sober up. However, as any alcoholic will tell you, sobering up is the really terrifying part of the addiction, and a major reason why alcoholism gets worse and problem drinkers keep drinking - I dreaded sobering up. Having normal hangovers for me, was now a long distant memory. The sort of hangover that normal people experience, when you have a headache and feel sick was a thing of the past. After living in my secret drinking existence for a few days, when I tried to sober up, the physical and emotional effects were terrifying. The sickness and diarrhoea lasted for a couple of days, to the point that I had to be near a toilet or I would have an accident, (which I sometimes did), and the stomach cramps, shaking and sweating were unlike anything I had ever experienced.

However it was the emotional symptoms, the absolute crippling anxiety and sheer panic, and the horrible feeling of impending doom that became increasingly impossible to bear. I felt like I could climb the walls and that I wanted to get out of my own skin – I just wouldn't know where to put myself I was so agitated and frightened. I also began to have really terrifying experiences in bed, when I would wake up and see spiders, sometimes big, sometimes small, but, to me, always absolutely real. I would literally be frozen with fear as they crept towards me or swarmed over the bed and walls.

I now know that what I was doing was very, very dangerous because of the risk of seizures and that every time I 'detoxed' myself I was taking a massive risk. Alcohol is one of the only drugs where withdrawal can cause death. This is why alcoholics undergoing treatment will have a medical detox, either in rehab or as an outpatient at home, with a medical professional overseeing their withdrawal. The fact that I was hallucinating about spiders frequently is a sign that I should have had medical help.

It will seem unbelievable to anyone reading this, but for a while I managed to live this way, even sobering up and appearing on QVC for five minutes with my business. Although, when this too failed in turning around the fortunes of my little company, it became yet another reason for me to wallow in self-pity.

Eventually, due to my fear of withdrawal, I began to sober up less and less, because I was terrified of how I would feel. When I had to see people, I would keep myself 'topped up' so that I had enough alcohol in my system to avoid withdrawal and basically get me through it, and when I didn't have to face anyone, I would drink until I passed out, wake up and start again.

This is especially heart breaking because my family and friends really thought that I was getting better and I am so sorry for deceiving everyone.

Having completed rehab for a second time and having one major relapse since then, (I say major because everyone knew about it, but there were many more stops and starts), my family knew I had been going to regular meetings and was doing the Twelve Steps with my Sponsor. But it was all now a sham. After spending a few months drinking after meetings and between them, now that Michael and Ross weren't around I had stopped going to meetings altogether, because they got in the way of drinking.

Communicating with people became a problem and I had to carefully plan phone calls. I would always try to keep a list of people I had spoken to on the phone, including Ross and Michael. After I had spoken to someone I would put a tick against their name if I felt that it had gone well and they hadn't suspected I was drunk. Eventually my writing was a scrawl and I couldn't read it, or I lost the list or just forgot to write one. That would send me into a blind panic the next day, but then I'd get drunk again and forget about it. Trying to maintain this kind of behaviour for a long period of time is, obviously, impossible and my relationships with those around me as well as my health began to deteriorate.

On top of the regular vomiting I had to go through before I could, eventually, hold down a drink every time I woke up, I had regular bouts of cystitis and conjunctivitis, which I am guessing were caused by dehydration. I can even remember dissolving sachets of cystitis relief medication into wine, which was probably the only time I actually used a glass to drink. Gross.

In fact my overall health was clearly deteriorating - my hair was falling out, my skin was grey and the dull ache in my side and my yellow looking bowel movements were a sign that my liver was suffering. It became normal for Ross to tell me that I needed to have a bath when he came home, and our weekends would often involve me staying in bed so that I could be near the bathroom toilet to vomit and have diarrhoea, because I had attempted not to drink to prepare for him coming home, but had mistimed my withdrawal.

During the week, when I was alone, I began to feel increasingly frightened. I would wake up in the middle of the night sweating, reach by the side of my bed and take a big swig from the bottle of wine that was always there, drinking it in the huge gulps that a person dying of thirst in the desert would take. I would then continue to drink until I fell asleep again, silently crying and feeling ashamed. In these moments I would think about how much I hated my life and what I had become and I would often think about killing myself, but, thankfully, never went through with it.

I don't know how the poor cat and dog must've felt. I would sometimes remember to feed them, but forget to let the dog out, (luckily the cat had a cat flap) and would sometimes be met with dog poo in the kitchen because the poor thing had been so desperate. I have met people over the years who had accidentally killed their beloved pets when they were drunk and could never forgive themselves or tell anyone the truth.

I also thought about rehab and AA and how I had failed, and how my drinking was now much worse than it had ever been, worse than I ever thought it could get.

I would think about Michael and how much I loved him, and how much I hated myself for putting him through things that no child should ever have to go through. At the same time I would also fantasise about being completely on my own and not needing anyone in my life, which would make it easier for me to just drink. Utter madness.

Going out for more supplies of wine was also difficult because I was usually over the limit to drive and would always promise myself that this would be the last time I would drive over the limit, but it never was. I had driven under the influence over the years, but now it was such a regular occurrence because I needed more and more alcohol. Sometimes I had to drive with one eye shut, just to try and focus. God only knows how I never crashed or killed someone. I am so ashamed of this period of my life that I find it very difficult to recount, but this is the reality of being a hopeless alcoholic who has reached rock bottom. You are going to die, it's as simple as that. If my life had continued like that for much longer, I would not be here.

As you descend into full blown, merciless, relentless alcoholism, accidents become more frequent and serious - falling over and splitting my head open, breaking ribs, falling on glass, (I still have a scar on my back, where I fell backwards into the bath onto a bottle of perfume which smashed, after being violently sick. The glass could've easily gone between my ribs and killed me). Alcoholics also have accidents in their car whilst drunk, maybe killing themselves and others, or they develop one of the many alcohol related illnesses and diseases. They also often take their own lives, because they cannot bear living in their alcoholic hell anymore.

In the dark, alone, I would think about dying, and how I would be remembered for being an alcoholic and nothing else. How my death, although sad, would probably be a relief to everyone, and how much I would miss everyone, especially my son and husband. I would think about how sorry I was, and resolve to stop drinking and seek help again. Then I would think about a life without alcohol, panic and reach for my wine bottle again, the dark shadow helping me because I was weak and shaking. Sometimes when I was too ill to make it to the toilet, I would vomit into a towel next to me on the bed and just lie there ashamed and crying. It was disgusting.

My life became completely consumed by alcohol and my absolute fear of sobering up completely, because of the withdrawal I would experience, and because of my inability to face people or confront what I now was. I was terrified of ever running out of alcohol, and even walked a couple of miles in the snow on a freezing night to buy wine. The wife that Ross had married was no longer there and he was coming back to a shell of a person – I can't imagine how he must've felt and again I am deeply sorry for what he had to go through.

When he was coming home, I would make sure that there was plenty of alcohol in all of my secret places – enough to see me through the weekend. An alcoholic without access to alcohol is vile and insufferable, and the knowledge that there were bottles dotted around the house to keep me topped up was essential to me. That's how I got through Christmas, in a fuzzy twilight world, permanently keeping a level of alcohol in my body from bottles hidden in wellingtons, under mattresses, rolled up in clothes in the wardrobe, and under bushes outside.

Then, after Christmas, when everyone had left and I was happily living my tragic, solitary existence, my secret world started to unravel. My niece Jenny rang me to tell me about a lovely surprise she was planning for my sister Eileen in a few months. I was so drunk that I had forgotten my own rule of never answering the phone when I was drunk. I can't remember our conversation, but I know that I was absolutely vile to her and basically told her what a terrible daughter she was. She is actually the most loving, funny, caring daughter you could ever meet. She was confused and hurt, but somehow I felt that I had probably done my sister a favour, and then I had some more to drink and passed out.

Waking up from that was horrific. The anxiety, the impending doom and the fear were all justified this time because I had been an utter cow, and I was frantic. I knew that I couldn't sort out the mess that I had created without admitting that I had been drinking. I realised that I couldn't stop drinking and would probably try to kill anyone who tried to stop me. This was far worse than I had ever imagined. I knew that I was unable to give up alcohol for anything and that it was killing me. I have never, ever been so afraid in my life.

I knew that I was killing myself, but that I didn't want to die. I didn't want to leave my son and husband and everyone who loved me. I didn't want to be this hideous, vile and, by now, smelly alcoholic. But nor could I face a life without alcohol. It had become the most important thing to me, and I was terrified of sobering up, of going through withdrawal and terrified of having to face the reality of my situation. There was a part of me that only wanted to be drunk and unconscious, and believed that was the only life that made any sense now - being sober was no-longer an option.

Everything I had read and been told about alcoholism had come true, and it had now reached a point where I couldn't live without it even if I wanted to, and all the while it was killing me and all of my relationships were disintegrating. I still couldn't believe this could have happened to me, and that I wasn't one of the three out of ten we had been told about in rehab who would survive this disease. I was simultaneously petrified of dying and wishing that I could die there and then to escape these feelings of desolation. I was finished.

Chapter 8

Finding Tim

In the February of 2015 I reached my 'rock bottom'. I had mainly been living alone as Ross was living in London Monday to Friday because of his promotion at work and Michael was at University. As usual, I had woken up in a half drunken haze but, unlike other mornings, when I reached down to the side of my bed, my wine bottle was empty.

After the initial disappointment and panic about whether I had any other bottles stashed around the house, I lay in bed in the still and silent house and just began to sob, because it hit me that this was how my life would be from now on until I died, which would be sooner rather than later. A secret, sad and lonely existence feeling ill and anxious when I was awake and drinking until I passed out again. In this respect my alcoholism was now very much a terminal illness. No human body can withstand an alcoholic's drinking indefinitely, and I was also taking extreme risks now every time I tried to 'self-detox' when I needed to sober up.

The house felt quiet and empty because Ross and Michael were effectively now gone and they were getting on with their lives. Thankfully for them, circumstances had taken them away from me and my drinking. Ross, who was too kind to actually leave me and end our marriage, was subtly moving on with his life and physically removing himself from me – simple self-preservation. Life goes on for other people – they don't just sit worrying about you because everyone has a limit to their patience and trust.

Now, what had been our lovely home was just a half packed up house full of hidden empty bottles and cans, inhabited by a hopeless and pathetic alcoholic whom they had both tried so often to help. It was my job to pack the house and get it ready for tenants who were going to rent it until we found a buyer, but with every day my timetable for packing and cleaning had to be amended because I would lose another day to drinking and / or being hungover.

I lay in bed and thought about how much I loved them, and how I ached to turn the clock back to be the mother I should've always been to Michael, the little boy I adored and who had shown me nothing but love. I was completely overwhelmed with sadness at the thought of not seeing him graduate, get a job, fall in love and get married, become a Dad...... I was going to miss him so much. But I knew that I was beaten.

I had been through rehab and AA and tried so many of my own ways to stop drinking, but now I simply couldn't face life without alcohol. I didn't even enjoy the taste, but I just couldn't bear to go through the horrendous withdrawal. I had no idea how I could ever even start to make amends with people – I simply couldn't face the thought of being sober.

This is when alcoholism often becomes a death sentence, because when you reach that point alcohol is probably going to kill you whether that be from a fall or accident, a car crash, suicide, one of the many alcohol related illnesses that alcoholics often develop, or a fatal seizure whilst trying to detox. I knew that in my case it would be from crashing my car, because when I needed to get more alcohol, all sense of right and wrong were forgotten.

Now even my car was full of empty miniatures of wine and squashed empty cans of gin and tonic. This is something that I am still deeply ashamed about, and I can barely even think about it without getting upset, because I know it was selfish and reckless. God only knows how I didn't kill or injure someone when I was at my worst.

I also knew then that when I moved south to be with Ross in just a matter of weeks, I wouldn't be able to hide how bad things were from him and that he wouldn't be able to cope. Recently, I felt that things that he had noticed recently were serious enough to bring about the end of our relationship, such as when he had to tell me that I needed to get a bath because I smelled. I knew that he would eventually leave me because no one should be expected to live like that. I couldn't stop drinking, so why should he have to stick around to watch me drink myself to death?

Fighting alcoholism is so tiring and draining. I had nothing left and had lost the battle. As I lay there accepting that my life was effectively over, I moved between wishing that I could die there and then, to being frightened of death, and back to just wanting it all to end because I was totally helpless and hated myself.

Physically, I wasn't able to lie there forever, because the awful panic and anxiety started to kick in which made me desperate for a drink. I hadn't planned properly and had no alcohol in the house. I paced around like an animal, not knowing where to put myself, unable to get my head straight, in order to plan what I was going to do. The anxiety that comes at this stage of alcoholism is so extreme that you literally want to crawl out of your own skin. Being inside your own body is unbearable and the only thing that can stop this it is having a drink.

This would usually be the point where I would have a swig of wine and start ringing people to 'check in', to make sure that they were still friendly to me, and that I hadn't upset anyone. Today I had no wine to give me the courage to do that, and I slowly remembered that I had upset my niece Jenny, my sister Eileen's daughter. I felt that familiar sick feeling of impending doom and blind panic that every alcoholic knows.

Standing in the middle of the dining room I cried out "please help me". I sobbed and sobbed, pacing the floor, and I tried frantically to contact Eileen and Jenny to beg forgiveness. Finally, I went to the computer on my desk and began searching the internet in desperation for someone or something to help me. I didn't know who or what, but I knew in that moment that if I got into the car and went to buy alcohol, that I would almost certainly have an accident. I also knew that I was losing everyone around me, and my self-destructive behaviour was accelerating out of control. Something within me forced me to have just one last attempt at getting help, which surprises me even now. I had done the same internet search so many times before, and wasted so much time and money on the people that I had found.

This is when I found Tim Phizackerley, who literally saved my life. Even though I had previously had such negative experiences with hypnotherapy, there was something about Tim's website that made me want to contact him. Someone must have been looking out for me that day, because Tim doesn't have the flashiest 'all singing all dancing' website to jump out at potential clients, but his warm smile in the photograph, and the fact that he is internationally renowned gave me that little flicker of hope that I had felt so many times before.

Tim has a list of problems and conditions that he can help with down the side of his page, and as soon as I saw alcohol that was good enough for me. Little did I know that the man with the friendly smile with the understated website would turn out to be a miracle worker.

I used the 'Contact Me' section on the website to send him a message and, because I was so upset and shaky, I simply wrote,

'I am an alcoholic who has tried everything including hypnosis'.

Reading this now is embarrassing, because it is more of a statement than a request for help and it probably came across as quite rude, as it seems like I simply couldn't be bothered to explain myself. I honestly think that I wrote it half hoping to get no response, so that I could throw my arms up and say 'I tried', and then carry on drinking. But the other half of me desperately wanted this man to instinctively know that I was so fragile and broken that my few words were a huge cry for help. Luckily for me, it was the latter and Tim simply replied,

'Hi Susan,
That doesn't surprise me one bit. And it doesn't bother me in the slightest either.
Remember that hypnosis is not a method: It is a tool. And tools give different results depending upon how skillfully they are used and in what way.
Not every woodworker can knock out a Chippendale chair for example. Not every painter can paint a Mona-Lisa. Abilities vary.
Why not give me a call and we can discuss it.
If I don't think I can help I will tell you.
Kind Regards, Tim'

These words still make me fill up with tears when I read them because they are so kind, disarmingly 'no nonsense' and reassuringly confident, without any drama or bravado, and not a hint of criticism towards other hypnotherapists. To me he seemed both professional and self-assured. No one could have blamed Tim if he had decided that he didn't want to waste his time on someone who didn't have the courtesy for a please or thank you, or even a simple explanation, but his reply was so warm and encouraging that I emailed him back immediately.

It all poured out: I was feeling desperate after yet another relapse, and I was also incredibly frightened because I felt that I had passed the point of no return.

We arranged to have a chat the following day, and although I managed to make the call, I must have sounded drunk because Tim reiterated several times that he couldn't help me unless I was sober when I saw him. Tim has a lovely, caring manner and I found it easy to be completely honest over the phone, (I had also realised that I had nothing to lose so there was no point in glossing over things). I practically begged him to help me, but he explained that he doesn't agree to see every person who contacts him because there are some people whom he knows instinctively will not respond to his approach.

So, in the first instance, he asked me to write everything I felt was relevant for him to know in an email, so that he could consider our telephone chat and my specific needs. Then he would decide if he could help me. I thought this was incredibly honest and even though cynics would point out that he could actually say that to everyone, there was just something about Tim that made me believe him.

I dutifully wrote my email immediately and sent it to him. I included everything I could about myself, because I wanted him to have every piece of information, whether it was relevant or not, right from my childhood through to the present sad situation I had created for myself. I so wanted him to agree to see me, and I desperately wanted to be able to give up drinking forever and get my life and Ross and Michael back. I can remember ending my email with the words –

'I don't want to die'.

After reading my email Tim agreed to see me which was an enormous relief. However, because he is very much in demand, he couldn't see me as soon as I would've hoped, and my appointment would have to be after I had moved out of our northern home to a rented house in the south. I knew that I had to face the prospect of another few weeks of out of control drinking, the risk of accident and upset, and the absolute certainty of self-loathing, shame and anxiety.

It's sad that this was just a matter of fact to me, but that was my reality by then. I couldn't even get excited about seeing Tim, because I knew that I had to hide and minimise the impact of my drinking over the next few weeks as I tried to prepare for the house move.

It's unthinkable to me now, and it must seem shocking to any non- alcoholic reading this, that during the short few weeks that I had to wait to see Tim, instead of trying to gradually wean myself off alcohol, I felt almost entitled to a few final blowouts.

The fact that Ross and Michael were lukewarm about my latest plan of action to get sober was sufficient ammunition for me to feel sorry for myself because no one trusted me.

Of course I never actually needed a real excuse to drink, and I spent the time alone before I had to move out of the house drinking and sleeping, packing bits of furniture and ornaments in a drunken haze. I know that this was my alcoholism's way of attempting to keep me close and sabotaging my last ditch attempt to get sober, and it almost worked because I became quite ill due to not eating properly. I lost a lot of weight, as my vomiting and diarrhoea became worse than ever, and had further bouts of cystitis and conjunctivitis.

While all of this was going on, my ability to run my business became, yet again, almost impossible. I think I must have phoned Jane in a drunken blind panic, because I can remember waking to find her crying next to my bed after I had yet again passed out. Jane was alarmed to see how skinny I had become, and got in touch with Eileen who had got in touch with Patricia.

All my sisters had their own lives and their own challenges to deal with, and I felt ashamed and angry with myself that, once again, I had become a cause for concern, despite my best efforts to keep myself to myself in my secret drinking world.

The game was up, yet again, and although I explained to them that it was all in hand and that I had booked an appointment with a guy called Tim, they had heard it all before and my sister Patricia came to stay at the house so that I couldn't drink.

Because no one knew how much I had been drinking and how bad things were by then, I had to endure the most horrible withdrawal, because I couldn't access any alcohol when she was there.

I can vividly remember having the most terrifying spider hallucinations, when I would lie in bed completely frozen with fear, watching them swarm over the bedding. Looking back, I know it was incredibly dangerous for me to do this without medical supervision, but my life was still such a lie that I felt I had no option other than to suffer in silence.

With the help of my sisters and then Ross, we packed the house and a rental van, and we made the first journey of my move south. Jane and her husband helped us this first time, which was just as well. I was supposed to be driving the van, but knew I was over the limit to do so. I didn't dare tell Ross, so I made an excuse about not being confident about driving such a large vehicle.

My brother in law offered to drive, and I went as a passenger with Ross in his car, making sure I had alcohol in my bag to drink when we stopped at the motorway services, (it is only recently that my brother in law told me that he suspected all along that I was drunk).

On our second and final journey, when I had to drive my own car from Newcastle to London, following Ross who had the cat and dog in his car, I knew that I had to put myself through withdrawal beforehand to be safe to drive the three hundred or so miles. As I have talked about before, I know now that my attempts to detox myself were very dangerous because of the risk of seizures which can't be predicted, but at the time I felt I had no option and tried to plan for the uncontrollable sickness and diarrhoea, and horrible spider hallucinations.

It was during this second journey that something happened that was like a huge slap in my self-destructive, alcoholic face. I like to imagine it was from my Guardian Angel who had watched on helplessly as I destroyed myself and now wanted to send me a message.

I had a blowout on the M1 which sent my car careering over all three lanes twice and, because my car was a tiny Smart Roadster, I believed for a few seconds that this was it. After all the drink driving I had done and outrageously got away with, I was now going to die sober, in my car, because of a blowout, (which was caused by a puncture from a screw, nail or some other debris in roadworks that I had recently driven through). I can remember trying to control my car, but expecting to be squashed by a lorry at any second and accepting that it was game over.

Somehow I managed to get the car onto the hard shoulder and immediately jumped out and stepped over the barrier at the side of the motorway. As I waited for the roadside assistance, I watched the hundreds of cars and lorries speeding past and the enormity of what had just happened consumed me. How I hadn't been hit by another vehicle when it was this busy as I swerved across the motorway in a car not much bigger than a go cart was nothing short of a miracle.

I knew that I wasn't meant to die then and felt overwhelmed with a realisation that I couldn't let myself die an alcoholic and waste this precious life that I had. Dramatic I know, but I simply couldn't believe how lucky I had just been, and when a lovely man who had been behind me and had seen the whole incident pulled in further up the hard shoulder and ran back to me with a high visibility top, he said exactly that. You are so lucky.

It only took a few hours (when I was safely in our new temporary home) for me to 'celebrate' my lucky escape with a drink of gin and tonic from the secret stash of cans hidden in a bag.

I followed this with another massive binge which started as a secret, but then became impossible to hide, and which left me incapable of going to a football match with Ross on our first proper weekend 'south' together. He had been looking forward to taking me to see his team and he was disgusted and angry. 'It's okay', I said, 'I'm seeing Tim next week'. He told me he honestly couldn't care less and went to the match with his friend. I knew then that I had no more chances with him – he was going to leave me.

And so the time came. After another self-detox followed by diarrhoea, sickness, cramps and spider hallucinations, I travelled back north to see Tim. I had arranged to stay at my sister Eileen's house the night before, so that I couldn't drink, because I knew that he couldn't help me if I was drunk, and I also knew that this had to work.

I thought a lot about the blowout on the motorway and how someone must be watching over me. I was so lucky to still be alive and yet I felt that I didn't deserve it. I was very nervous to see Tim, which I had fully expected to be, but I was also worried that I didn't feel excited or hopeful at all – I had a horrible feeling deep down that I was a hopeless case and that this would be another waste of time and money. I wanted it to work, but I knew now that I was dealing with something that was so much more powerful than I had ever imagined, and it had me in a grip that I had never believed possible. The realisation that I would die if this didn't work was quite unbearable and I felt sick and emotional.

When I arrived at Tim's office he immediately put me at ease and I felt incredibly safe and relaxed, and allowed myself to believe, for the time that I was with him, that he really could help me.

Tim explained very carefully what we were going to do and why, in a way that I could understand. He has a vast knowledge of the workings of the mind, but is able to talk about the most complex things using very relatable analogies. I could tell instantly that he genuinely cares about the people that he sees and wants them to be free of whatever problems they might have that have brought them to him.

I have mentioned before that I believe the vast majority of alcoholics will have some idea as to what might have caused them to become an alcoholic. Even if they can't pinpoint one thing, there will be underlying issues that they know they need to address, which they may have already talked about during NHS counselling sessions, at AA or in rehab. Through reading my email, chatting to me on the telephone and talking to me face to face in his office that day, Tim was able to create a completely personal session, totally unique and specific to me and my needs, and where, surprisingly, alcohol was addressed towards the end of the long day. There were also beliefs that I had about myself deep down in my subconscious that I wasn't aware of, which triggered certain behaviours, which we also gradually uncovered and worked on.

Over the course of the one and only day that I spent with Tim, he combined an intensive, (and exhausting), mix of hypnosis, regression and percussive suggestion tools, (PSTEC), interspersed with talking and lots of his unique wisdom and common sense, to gradually uncover, unravel and extinguish one by one every issue which had underpinned my alcoholism. He quite simply made each misguided belief, destructive emotion and deeply upsetting memory completely disappear for me forever, and when he had done that, right at the end of the day, he destroyed any desire for alcohol and the hold that it had had over me. He crushed and terminated my dark shadow and it simply vanished.

I had done enough talking about myself and my drinking over the years to develop my own theories about why I drank. I had poured this out in my email to Tim, but he was able to unearth important missing pieces, which completed the puzzle, and which had been holding me back and perpetuating my cycle of self-destructive behaviour for years. He did this through regression techniques, using hypnosis to take me back to certain events and situations that I had chosen to forget. Some memories sit deep inside our subconscious and we cannot recall them because they are 'repressed', but they can still have a profound impact on our lives in spite of that. Regression can guide us back so that we can access those events and then address them and the impact that they might be having on our behaviour.

Once we had a negative belief or memory that we could work on, Tim then used a tool called PSTEC, something which he invented and created based on years of experience working with the mind. PSTEC has been described as being 'possibly the fastest and most efficient way to neutralise problem emotions ever created'. It uses a unique audio track and tapping and he developed it to make otherwise difficult things much faster and simpler to achieve.

Tim then dealt with all of my issues, one by one and, no matter how trivial they might seem to someone else, he effectively extinguished my deep rooted insecurities and dismantled all of my emotional baggage bit by bit. I think it would be very useful here to use one of my own examples, which we addressed that day. Although this was one of the less serious issues, it was very emotional for me and we discovered in my session with Tim that it was still having a profound effect on how I reacted to events and people years later.

When I entered senior school, and between the ages of twelve and fourteen, I was one of the many pupils in the school who received free school meals. The system that they had in place was, I still believe, very cruel in that in order to receive a free meal, you had to present a pass with your name on it. The passes were spread out on a dining table in a corner of the dining room, but you could only access the table once you had been in the dining queue with your friends for a while, because of the layout of the area.

Therefore, every single lunchtime, I was required to leave my friends and go to the table in full view of everyone to search for my pass and then re-join the queue. The problem was, the passes were thrown in a heap on the table, no alphabetical order to speed things up, so I often spent what seemed like an age frantically searching for my pass, as my friends continued moving ahead in the queue.

I would be crimson with embarrassment because at that age appearance is everything, there was probably some boy that I fancied watching, my hormones were all over the place.... It was just a really humiliating experience, and unnecessarily so.

This sounds trivial, but I know that I was always quick to feel inferior throughout my life, or believe that people were looking down on me when they weren't, (even friends). I understand now that this was not real, but for years the slightest comment or unexpected situation could transport me back to the excruciating feeling of the lunch queue at school.

With Tim's PSTEC, I was required to listen to an audio which contained his voice, as well as different tones which I was required to tap in time to. I had to listen and tap as well as feel the feeling that I wanted to extinguish as intensely as possible, (in this example, the embarrassment and feeling of being 'poor').

Gradually, trying to concentrate on everything at once - Tim's voice, the tones, the tapping and the feeling - was just too much, and ultimately the feeling disappeared as I tried to tap with the tones.

Over several hours, Tim eliminated my worries and anxieties one by one and he cleared the way in order for him to find and reinforce the positive things about me that I had lost along the way. Then, most importantly for me, he dealt with my relationship with alcohol using PSTEC. He placed a bottle of white wine in front of me and said I had to feel the desire for it as strongly as possible- which was not difficult. I then followed the PSTEC instructions and extinguished completely any craving or yearning for alcohol – forever.

I am not an expert on hypnotherapy, regression or PSTEC, (and my recollection of the day is, understandably hazy), so I asked Tim to sum up his approach in his own words – and he does this so much better than me. This is what he said –

"First I look to eliminate any distorted disempowering beliefs and crushing negative emotions. And because it's important and because I'm dealing with a person who initially can't see the truth for themselves, I look for all the wonderful in them and all the good that should be revealed to them ... and also their unique strengths and potential. So I then use hypnosis and other tools to help them see and experience those things for themselves. It's not rocket science. It's mostly a matter of one person genuinely caring about the other person and then doing things in the correct way using the right tools in the right order. It's a partnership with a very specific intended outcome."

"My approach to treating an alcohol "addiction" may seem somewhat strange to someone unfamiliar with my way of thinking, but most of the time it does seem to work very well so I would say I'm on the right track. My attitude going in is that what appears to be an "addiction" is not an addiction at all. It may absolutely seem like one but it isn't. Instead an alcohol "addiction" is a symptom of a very different problem altogether ...and that problem is typically a long lasting, deep or unresolved unhappiness.

Such a deep unhappiness typically revolves around sets of very negative beliefs about self. These beliefs seem utterly real to their unfortunate owners and hence life has often seemed hopeless to any person who has those beliefs. Such beliefs are guaranteed to relate to past events and have almost always been made worse by guilt surrounding alcohol and the excessive drinking. Toxic beliefs typically create awfully dark associated emotions.

Alcohol then is typically being used by the person either as the means to seek some kind of escape or sometimes as a form of unwitting self-punishment. Added to that are the other usual mistaken beliefs. Examples are that the problem is unsolvable, or that it is a kind of chemical addiction (even though it isn't). There are often also very unhelpful beliefs about having a disease or of having an addictive personality. Such beliefs are not helpful in the slightest. They make a person feel powerless and imprisoned. There's a habit element too. The habit element forms over time and certain things will also typically have become triggers. I generally have to sweep away all of these and many other unhelpful beliefs which would otherwise cause problems in treatment.

Of course I also look to identify the original reasons for the long lasting unhappiness. Then by using a variety of methods (hypnosis included) I set about correcting all of those things one at a time. Although this sounds very time consuming, the truth is that with practice and with the right methods this can often be done quite quickly.

There's more though, because from the very first moment and throughout our time together, I'm also looking to identify all of a person's real strengths and also looking to locate their great or truly wonderful qualities. This is because I want my client to see and feel those good things deeply in themselves too! I want them to get a powerful sense of their own genuine huge value and tremendous potential. Being a hypnotist is extremely helpful in allowing me to help someone to finally see these things for themselves.

With all of this done I can then at last address alcohol itself which by this point in time is almost an afterthought.

My biggest frustration though is that other therapists aren't doing this and why not? It's not rocket science. It's mostly common sense and usually it works. It simply needs to be done well and correctly."

Because Tim combines several approaches in one session, I would say that hypnotherapy is too narrow a definition of what Tim practices. Although he is also a hypnotherapist and a hypnotist, PSTEC and hypnosis are very different indeed, and in his own work he uses both. As I said, it was a long and exhausting day, uncovering things that I hidden away deep in my subconscious and then making them irrelevant.

He completely re-wired my brain and turned very deep rooted negative beliefs into something incredibly positive – and overwhelmingly powerful, and he extinguished thoughts of alcohol forever. In my opinion hypnotherapy on its own cannot cure alcoholism, and the hypnotherapists that I had met over the years were even less likely of success, because they hadn't even delved into my background or back story. However, the results of Tim's unique combination of approaches, in my own simple terms, was like a miracle.

And it was done in one session.

I realise that many people will have a problem believing that one session with Tim effectively 'cured' me of my alcoholism, and I understand that completely, so I want to spend time explaining why I believe Tim's approach worked based on all of my experiences with AA, rehab, Counselling and other hypnotherapists.

I know that if I had just stopped drinking, the problems and deep rooted emotional issues that I had would still be there, so it is essential and correct that they had to be addressed and dealt with, but it is also refreshing and so liberating that they have been erased completely. As the old saying goes, if you want to heal a wound, stop touching it, but isn't that what we do over and over again in AA and counselling? We keep on re-visiting and touching old wounds, so that they can never heal and we give energy to our alcoholism by talking about it all of the time.

This is so important for me to stress because, in the world of AA and rehab, labels such as 'dry drunk' are used to describe alcoholics who are not drinking, but who are not 'sober', because they still have lots of unresolved issues that they are battling with. There is a belief that you cannot be genuinely sober if you have not dealt with problems from your past or your 'character faults', but traditionally, this can take a long time.

As I mentioned in Chapter 4, I strongly believe that an alcoholic does not have the luxury of time to devote to talking about problems week after week, (during counselling), because the alcohol is still there, depressing them and taking them further down the spiral in between counselling sessions. I again must stress here that I understand that counselling is an essential lifeline for many people, but this is about my alcoholism and for me, talking whilst still drinking had proven futile in the past.

This also brings me to the belief in Alcoholics Anonymous, that only alcoholics can help alcoholics. Tim Phizackerley has never been an alcoholic, and he didn't need to understand the behaviours specific to an alcoholic to stop me from drinking, he just understands that any destructive behaviour has a cause that can be switched off, and once that is done, the destructive behaviour can then be switched off too - permanently. The gaps in the subconscious that the negative beliefs and issues leave can then be filled with positivity and confidence to create a new future which starts then and there, in my case without alcohol. To put it simply, he stopped my negative beliefs and feelings about myself, stopped any desire for alcohol, and reinforced the positives about myself which had always been there but that I had lost along the way.

I have heard that there is no scientific study which shows that hypnotherapy has a place in the treatment of alcoholics and my experience with the five hypnotherapists that I saw over the years would be proof for most people that this is true. However, as I have stressed, hypnotherapy is only one element of Tim's approach. I believe that I am proof (along with all of the other alcoholics that Tim has helped), that he has developed a treatment that saves lives, and takes away the daily exhausting struggle of using willpower to resist picking up a drink.

As with any hypnotherapy, when you wake up, you don't know whether or not it has worked. Only time would tell, but I left the office feeling a warm glow of hope, unaware at that point that effectively, a miracle had just occurred. I thought of how I had imagined my dark shadow while I listened to Tim's voice and the tones, and had made myself feel the desire for alcohol as I had looked at the white wine bottle. I had tapped and tapped the dark shadow away. It got smaller and smaller, squeaked pathetically and then it was gone.

Chapter 9

Learning To Be Sober – Life After Tim

Unlike some of my other attempts at getting sober, there was no fanfare or fuss around my meeting with Tim. I was embarrassed to talk about it to anyone, to be honest, because I had built everyone's hopes up so often in the past. I'd made what seemed like a million promises and had so often broken them. I also sensed that everyone had moved on with their lives and distanced themselves from me emotionally – a kind of self-preservation and I really didn't blame them. My sense of guilt and shame told me that they were no longer interested in the same old story and my broken promises, and that they were beginning to accept that the old Susan would never be back.

I left my session with Tim feeling very relaxed, but not knowing whether seeing him had worked for me or not – that would only become apparent over time, which is true of any treatment for alcoholism. I had arranged to meet Michael before I drove back south and I was very nervous to see him. I knew that he, like Ross, had put up an invisible barrier as far as I was concerned, in order to protect himself and to be able to get on with his own life.

I had put them both through so much, especially over the last two years and he was happily enjoying his new life at university. Both Ross and Michael could be forgiven for taking my latest attempt at 'sorting myself out' with a pinch of salt, because I had promised so many times that 'this time things would be different'.

It is tragic really, because every time I saw a new hypnotherapist or counsellor, started attending AA meetings or went into rehab I really did believe that this time I was going to be able to stop drinking, and my determination and enthusiasm had managed to convince Michael and Ross and the people who loved me to believe in me – for a while. However they had given up believing in me a long time ago and it's understandable that those close to an alcoholic can feel that they have been made a fool of after putting their faith in the person and supporting them again and again.

So when I met Michael, I wasn't expecting any great excitement or even enthusiasm around my latest endeavour to stop drinking, I just desperately wanted to see him and tell him that I was sorry. However, I had the sense not to do that because, again, he had heard it all before. So we met for some food at a pub near to his Dad's house, (he had coincidentally been visiting Mark), and I explained in a factual way about my meeting with Tim and what we had done that day and he simply said, 'well, I hope for your sake that it has worked'.

I so desperately wanted to cuddle him and beg him to believe that he was the most important thing in my life, and that the alcoholic me wasn't the real me, but I resisted doing that – I knew I had pushed him too far and that I had to allow time to not only prove that I wasn't drinking, but to hopefully heal the damage that I had done.

The same was true of Ross. I knew that he was beyond fed up with the life that I was giving him and he would have left me by then if his job hadn't forced us to be apart and given him an escape. If he'd still been living with me full time, he would have realised how hopeless things had become and would've been sucked deeper into the chaos and destruction that my drinking caused and the hurt and embarrassment that comes with that.

Now that I too had moved south, I knew that if my drinking continued and Ross had to endure my alcoholic existence 24/7, he would definitely leave me before drinking killed me, because no person can or should be expected to live that life. No matter how much someone has loved you in the past, you cannot stay 'in love' with an alcoholic, because it robs them of their real personality and the qualities that made them attractive. All you're left with is this dishevelled, aggressive and frequently incontinent shell of a person. Who should be expected to stay with that? The life with me that he had found exciting in the beginning because it was 'never boring' was now very boring – and tragic.

So, as I drove down the M1 to my new life in London, I decided that, no matter what happened in the future, if I wasn't drinking, no day from now on could ever be as bad as the last time I'd felt the crippling anxiety of withdrawal, or the blind panic of running out of alcohol. I was here now despite reaching rock bottom. I had survived those days and I decided I could face anything if I wasn't drinking, no matter how bad – after all, if I stayed sober I couldn't make my life any worse than it was now.

I decided that I wasn't going to rush anything or anyone, myself included, and that I was going to simply 'be', without any expectations, excitement, big plans or forced attempts to make things better. I decided to take a step back and 'cocoon' myself for a while. I had spent so long causing so much chaos, worry, anger and disappointment, that I needed to allow the dust to settle and those around me to get on with a normal life. This gave time for Tim's words to work on my subconscious and allow me to be open to whatever life now had in store for me. You could say that I completely 'surrendered' myself, because I had nowhere else to go. In that respect there had already been a subtle but profound shift in my behaviour, which I didn't realise then.

Now this is all very good in theory, but the reality was very hard, mainly because my mind and emotions were delicate and raw to say the least. The 'naked' vulnerability I had felt after rehab all that time ago was there again, but this time probably multiplied by a hundred. This is difficult to explain, but I will try my best!

When you give up drinking after being in rehab or attending AA meetings, alcohol is still there and your dark shadow still wants to convince you to drink. You're still using 'willpower' and whatever strength you can muster to stop yourself from drinking, so a lot of your subconscious and conscious thoughts are still revolving around drinking- wanting alcohol, resisting alcohol, hating alcohol, missing alcohol…. (especially if you're attending AA meetings, because you are talking about it all of the time).

It's like splitting up from someone who you are madly in love with, but you know is really bad for you because your relationship is toxic. It's the right thing to do, but it takes a while to get them from under your skin.

I noticed very quickly that alcohol never entered my mind from the day that I saw Tim, but I only realised this when I reminded myself to count the days since I'd had a drink because, miraculously, alcohol had ceased to mean anything to me or have any place in my thoughts.

Because of this, there was this enormous 'space' that used to be filled by my alcoholic thinking - my self-loathing, guilt, temptation, cravings, shame, the battle that goes on 24/7 for an alcoholic when you are trying not to pick up a drink.

The enormous amounts of energy that my inner battle must have consumed over the years was such a complete waste of my life, and I think this might explain why so many alcoholics pick up again after rehab or while attending AA meetings - they are simply exhausted because alcohol continues to creep into their thoughts and wear them down.

So now I had this 'void' where my alcoholic thoughts used to exist, and my mind filled it with all sorts of things that now seem very sad and odd, but were very confusing and alarming, at the same time as being important to me at the time. Again, this is difficult to explain, because my mind was, quite frankly, all over the place.

I was realistic enough not to expect to suddenly have absolute mental clarity and the kind of rational, normal everyday thoughts that everyone takes for granted, because it is simply a biological/physiological fact that it can take an alcoholic's brain years to recover. I was by now an expert on alcoholism and recovery because of all of the reading that I had done over the years, and I was well aware of the probable damage that I had done, not only to my body but also my brain and thought processes, emotions and memory.

One of the many phrases that I use to try to explain my alcoholism is 'self-inflicted dementia' and I was very worried about the impact that my years of alcohol abuse might have had on my 'mind', but I also knew that only time would tell if that was the case. In the meantime, I spent a lot of time in the first few weeks thinking about death and mortality, which may seem strange because by stopping drinking I was hoping to avoid dying at a relatively young age.

It was like waking up from a long sleep, and I kept thinking, this is it, this is my life, but where do I start? I felt completely lost and afraid that I had wasted so many years and that I couldn't possibly begin to even try to make up for lost time – and that because I was now middle aged I would soon be dead. I had almost completely obliterated my forties with alcohol and I was so scared – scared of never making up for lost time or doing anything with my life before I died.

But mostly, I was very scared that Michael and Ross wouldn't be able to love me. They had moved on emotionally for their own self-preservation, and I didn't know if they could ever trust me or even like me again, but I also knew that I had no right to expect anything from them.

So, the old familiar feelings of worthlessness, hopelessness and failure were back and this time with a huge amount of regret and fear added in. But, instead of turning to alcohol and drinking these unbearable and crippling emotions away, I instead became increasingly aware of a calm and reassuring but tiny voice in the background, telling me that these feelings wouldn't last forever – this too shall pass.

The understanding that had come to me during the drive down the M1 after seeing Tim would wash over me again and again – that no matter how bad I felt now, no feeling could ever be as bad as the gut wrenching shame and impending doom that I used to wake up with after drinking.

It would only come to me much further down the line what a blessing this 'void' in my life was, and still is, and all of the amazing things that I could potentially achieve with the enormous amounts of emotional energy that had been released by seeing Tim. Energy that, in the past, I had wasted day after day, thinking about alcohol and drinking.

The same energy used by so many recovering alcoholics all over the world who are using willpower and inner strength day in day out to not have a drink and to simply survive, whilst they are attending AA or trying to remain sober on their own, had been gifted back to me.

Tim had released me from a lifetime of struggling and battling with that constant, draining temptation which is the price most alcoholics have to pay for sobriety, and he had given me the gift of complete freedom from even the thought of alcohol. I still cannot quite believe this but I am more than happy to accept it and not over analyse it. I just know that I am so lucky to have found him and I am grateful every day.

However it would be a good while before I could even begin to think about the bigger picture and, in the immediate aftermath of my meeting with Tim, my main focus was on simply trying to start again and be 'normal'. I decided that I would be patient with myself and try to be kind, and not dwell on the lost years and horrible things that I had done.

I didn't ever expect kindness from anyone else, but I knew that no amount of shame, guilt or regret could ever get the wasted years back. Even now, although I believe that It's a good thing that I still have regrets and guilt, and can remember how wretched I felt when I was drinking, I don't let these feelings rule my life or make me hate myself.

There are still plenty of reminders that pop up from time to time. For example, Ross might talk about an event that we attended or a gig that we were at while I was drinking, and he's surprised when and I simply cannot remember it at all, because he didn't realise at the time that I was drunk.

I cannot remember seeing George Michael -who I absolutely loved - because of an alcohol induced blackout. Unbelievable and shameful for me now, but that's how bad some of the gaps in my memory are, and there are regretfully many events and trips that are hazy or forgotten.

This is something that I have to learn to live with, but it still makes me sad. Worse than that, there are also friends and acquaintances from my past that are now gone from my life forever, because of my drunken behaviour, which is so much worse and much more difficult to come to terms with.

Once I had accepted that I could never turn back the clock and made the decision to try to look forward and be patient with myself, as well as deciding I should have zero expectations of forgiveness or faith in me from anyone, I turned my attention to more pressing practical matters, such as getting a job.

From a purely financial point of view, we needed the money because a move from the North East to the South of England is not cheap and it was a monetary shock to the system. My business wasn't even paying off its debts and even I had to accept, in my new sober state, that it wasn't ever going to be the success I had dreamed it would be all those years before.

As well as being frustrated with my drinking Ross was, understandably, frustrated that he had supported me all of this time with my invention, and I knew that I had to begin to contribute to our new life in the south.

This created a new dilemma for me because my years of drinking had left me unsure as to what I had ever been good at. I honestly didn't know what my brain was capable of anymore and whether the alcohol abuse had depleted my intelligence or ability to make quick decisions, solve problems or whether I could cope in a work environment. Trying to articulate this to Ross came across as self-pitying and selfish, and I knew that he had already been pushed further than most partners would have tolerated and was probably still expecting me to start secretly drinking again.

So I went through a period where I quietly applied for random jobs which were totally inappropriate considering my fragile state at that time and which even now would be completely unsuitable because of my lack of experience and my personality type - these included applying to MI5 to be involved in intelligence work, several presenting jobs on shopping channels because of my five minutes on QVC, the Head of Marketing for a large pharmaceutical company, Researcher in the House of Commons…. If it wasn't so sad it would be funny.

At the time I can remember becoming increasingly panicked because I wanted to make Ross and Michael proud of me again, but I'd been out of the workplace for so long and I began to believe that no one would employ an out of touch and middle aged recovering alcoholic.

Again, in the past this kind of defeatist, self-pity would be enough to sabotage any attempts at staying sober and given me an excuse to pick up a drink. But now there was something there stopping me from even thinking about drinking, and spurring me on to try to get my life back and rebuild my relationships with Michael and Ross.

I know now that Tim had tapped into the inner strength that must have always been inside me, as well as giving me back the confidence in myself that I had lost along the way. The old Susan was gradually returning, but at the time I simply took each day as it came and tried to be the best that I could be and quietly get on with things. No fuss and no drama after years of exactly that.

From a practical point of view, I found a fantastic organisation set up specifically to help women of similar age to me who were looking to re-enter the workplace after a long period away. With their help I updated my CV and managed to tailor my job search to more appropriate and realistic positions.

From an emotional point of view, my resolve not to rush Ross and Michael and to try to be a normal wife and mother was more difficult, and there were times when I expected too much and tried too hard. I would end up crying and then beg for forgiveness and felt like I could never get the balance right.

But every time I felt desperately sad and believed I'd ruined everything and could never fix it, I would remind myself that even if this was as good as it ever got, no feeling would ever be as bad as the feelings I had after drinking – this too shall pass.

There were some very dark times when I felt incredibly low, sorry and full of regret and fear that I had lost the love of Michael and Ross forever, but I somehow managed to resist making a big deal of this to them and, more importantly, I never thought about drinking those feelings away. I decided to write down my feelings and fears instead of spilling them out and sharing them with anyone else, so that I could attempt to process them and not burden anyone with the torment and desperate panic that I was experiencing.

For a long time I thought Michael no longer wanted me in his life, and during that time I would visit him at university, trying so hard not to cry. This period of my diary has been very difficult for me to read again and is too private to share. Suffice to say that I was frequently in complete meltdown over the damage I had done to our relationship, but I knew that to burden Michael with that would've been selfish and even more destructive.

I am telling you all of this, because it's important that I am honest about the reality of emerging from alcoholism, feeling naked and vulnerable. I was learning how to be a 'whole' person again and, early on, I sometimes felt very lost. However it also proves to me the life changing power of my session with Tim and the strength it gave me which had a profound effect on my previous knee jerk reactions to difficult situations.

I'd spent so many years blotting everything out with alcohol numbing every feeling, good and bad, and now I was dealing with the terrifying possibility that I may have lost the respect and love of my husband and son forever, but I never once wanted to drink. I understood that you cannot spend years spiralling into alcoholism and then existing as a hopeless alcoholic without causing immense hurt and embarrassment to those closest to you, so I couldn't expect anyone to believe that my session with Tim had miraculously worked or to welcome me with open arms and forget everything that had happened.

I had to keep this in mind and endure the fear that I might not ever be able to get their respect and trust back and I also had to allow myself time to 'evolve' back into being the real me again. So I kept waking up each day and just being grateful that I wasn't drinking and that Ross still lived with me and Michael still wanted to meet me sometimes.

Slowly, as Ross began to notice that I wasn't tempted to numb my feelings with alcohol, our relationship began to improve as he gradually allowed himself to believe that my session with Tim had been worthwhile. My meetings with Michael also began to become less intense over time. I was able to relax and allow myself to simply be his Mum and very slowly I started to regain my confidence. I allowed myself to believe that I could be a loving - and loved - wife and mother again, and maybe even a fun person to be around further down the line.

Remarkably, during all of that time while the fears and doubts about getting my life and the love of Ross and Michael back, (as well as the respect of my family and friends), were whirring around in my head, there was one thing that I was always absolutely certain of from the day that I saw Tim. I knew that I would never drink again.

I just knew alcohol would never again be important to me, however I knew better than to actually say this to anyone because it was just too enormous a statement to make after all of the false promises I had made before. I understood that I simply had to allow time to prove that I was sober and that I was not tempted by alcohol and, at the same time, try to be a wife and a mother and earn a living. But secretly I began to feel more and more excited because I knew that, thanks to Tim, I had escaped alcohol forever - it was that simple.

I had absolute confidence in the fact that I would never have to waste energy fighting temptation and cravings ever again, or need to attend AA meetings for the rest of my life, and I wanted to shout it from the rooftops because I was so certain - and I still am.

Paradoxically, in spite of that absolute belief, (which has only strengthened over time), I knew that if I ever did have a drink again, I wouldn't want to stop until I was completely drunk. To me this is evidence of the enormous shift in my thinking and behaviour that my session with Tim has brought about.

In the past when I had periods of abstinence, there was always that belief and hope in the back of my mind that one day I would be able to drink normally again, and the false sense of security that comes with an extended period of not drinking is what alcohol uses to seduce the alcoholic into taking their first drink again. Now I am under no illusions and I know that I can never, ever drink alcohol normally, and this simple acceptance and honesty with myself is completely of Tim's making and something which I had always been reluctant to admit or even entertain in the past.

Because I now accept this one hundred percent, even though I know that I will never drink again, I would never under any circumstances test it. Like I said, this seems paradoxical and is difficult for me to understand but, as with many of the changes that Tim has brought about in my life, I don't over analyse it or question it. I talk about this in more detail in Chapter 10 (when I look at practical tips around drinking and socialising), but suffice to say, I am incredibly protective of my sobriety and, in spite of the fact that I never even notice or think about alcohol now, I wouldn't be stupid enough to risk allowing alcohol to enter my mouth. I know now that I never drank in the past because I liked the taste or because a certain wine complemented a certain food - I always drank alcohol for the affect it had on my feelings and confidence, and then I eventually drank with the sole aim of getting drunk. I know that if I drank now, that reality would not have changed and I would start where I left off and eventually kill myself with alcohol.

So, from the day I met Tim, I had a tiny flicker of excitement and confidence that I was 'cured' and wouldn't drink again mixed with the fear of never being able to repair the damage that I had done to relationships, as well as the confusion and worry from a practical point of view of 'Where do I start? What is my brain capable of? What am I good at?'.

I had moved on from my tendency to randomly apply for the most inappropriate and unsuitable jobs, mainly with the help of the careers organisation that I had found who had helped me to think seriously about what I could genuinely offer to an employer, but my main concern was that I had probably damaged my brain and would not be able to keep up in any job or workplace. I persevered and secured an interview, my first in years, and eventually began working again in a customer services / order processing role for an online retailer. I continued my journey towards a 'normal' existence and, although I knew that this job was never going to be something that I wanted to do long term, it was an important boost to my confidence and a vital learning experience.

In day to day life, there were obviously countless 'first times' for doing things completely sober such as dancing, having an argument, attending a party, Christmas – the list is endless. Some things were more challenging than others, especially dancing because when I'd had a drink I always imagined that I had impressive moves on the dancefloor and great rhythm, (I think that most of us do), but stone cold sober it took me a while to loosen up, but again I persevered!

Over time the enormous gift of freedom from alcohol that Tim had given me and the incredible escape that I had had, began to become increasingly evident, not only to me, but to those closest to me – my family and the friends who hadn't deserted me.

I am blessed with such wonderful family and friends, and one thing they certainly know how to do well is to enjoy themselves and party, but I had always found social gatherings difficult if I was going through a period of abstinence in the past. Inevitably, if I found myself in a situation where people were drinking I would feel uptight and uncomfortable and, more importantly, resentful of them, that I would end up stealing drinks and downing them secretly to relax.

Because of this, the only real solution was to avoid being around alcohol at all and to avoid these events completely. This is, sadly, a reality that many alcoholics find themselves in, and they have to either avoid everyday happy occasions and celebrations all together, even something as innocent as a Christening, or they have to muster all the strength and willpower they can to get themselves through simply being there.

This focus and mental battle with temptation and triggers not only means that an alcoholic can't relax and enjoy themselves, but it's also very emotionally draining. When I found myself in situations like that in the past, it made me hate myself for being so weak and 'different', and wishing that I could drink normally - that is when alcohol whispers to the alcoholic and convinces them that 'a couple of glasses won't hurt'.

The amazing gift of complete freedom from any thoughts of alcohol that Tim had given to me came as an unexpected surprise. When I had contacted him desperate for him to help me and for me to stop drinking, my goal had been to stay alive because I knew that alcohol was killing me, but I just couldn't stop drinking.

Being able to attend parties surrounded by people who are drinking and enjoying themselves or even being a hostess and pouring drinks for others never even crossed my mind back then. In fact, it's an obvious piece of advice in AA and rehab, and a way of life which most recovering alcoholics adopt and that is, if at all possible, to avoid situations involving alcohol. This makes complete sense and I would never have deliberately sought to test this out. My main focus was to repair my relationships and to live the best life I could.

But gradually, I realised that I didn't even notice when people were drinking! Where previously I would've clocked every drink in the room, every sip people took and every opportunity to sneak a drink, now I just enjoyed the company of my friends and family and didn't register the alcohol. It was nothing short of a miracle and my friends, who were at first cautious and awkward about drinking around me, were staggered when they realised that being around alcohol didn't bother me at all.

Only an alcoholic will understand how amazing this freedom must feel and, believe it or not, this is where other alcoholics that I have spoken to have problems believing the complete 'switch off' in my brain. They think it's just too good to be true because of the internal battles they fight, but for me it's a happy fact of life. Just imagine the complete freedom and joy of being able to enjoy everything that your friends and family do, without worrying about temptation or triggers? Imagine dancing and partying and having friends for dinner and pouring wine, without ever being tempted to drink or even noticing alcohol? That is what Tim gave to me – a very happy added bonus on top of saving me from alcohol.

Ross and Michael like to share a beer and don't have to worry about me being tempted or feel guilty about drinking around me. Our friends Gayle and Jason host the most fun, late into the night, dance until you drop parties, and I am always there until the end, enjoying every moment and laughing and dancing with Ross and Michael. My wonderful siblings, nieces and nephews love to party and the three of us are there in the thick of it. No one I'm close to needs to alter their behaviour around me, which is a real blessing for me. They don't feel guilty about drinking and I don't have the guilt or worry that comes with needing people to behave differently around me because I'm teetotal.

However the most important thing to me after seeing Tim was, and still is, fixing my relationships with Michael, Ross and my family and friends, as well as trying to live a good life and be the best version of me that I can be. After I left Tim's office, I never expected anything from anyone because I had caused so much hurt and chaos, and from that moment I somehow had the wisdom to be patient and not to rush things. First I had to start unpicking the years of 'muddle' in my head that alcohol had caused and understand how this may have affected my opinion of myself and how I interacted with people - both good and bad.

One thing that I did learn from AA and rehab is that most alcoholics, myself included, are 'people pleasers', and I also recognised that while I was drinking I was always on the 'back foot' - always feeling guilty and ashamed and ready to blame myself for everything whether it was my fault or not, which might not necessarily bring out the best behaviour in some people. I needed to start to allow my true personality to come through and, as well as making amends for the bad things that I had done, I needed to get some self-respect back, before I could expect others to respect me.

This is an ongoing process and the confidence that Tim reignited in me back then has steadily grown over time, helping me to withstand knocks along the way and have faith in time being a healer. Starting back then with baby steps, and that fear of not knowing who I was or if I could ever imagine Michael and Ross forgiving me and loving me, I have slowly re-discovered the good in myself and worked to rebuild my relationships with people. One of the very valuable lessons that I have taken from AA is that you should only ever try to make amends with people if it will not hurt them more by doing so. I have respected this and accepted that there are some people who wouldn't want to hear from me again. It is heart-breaking for me that some of my relationships didn't survive my drinking over the years, but that is the reality of alcoholism – it destroys love and friendships.

For a long time after I met Tim, while I was trying to shake off the people pleasing aspect of my alcoholic existence and regain some self-respect, it was often difficult to get the balance right, for example, between assertiveness and aggression! Because I wasn't used to being assertive unless I'd had a drink, (when I would become aggressive), it was difficult for me and I liken it to someone who has received a bionic hand and is learning how to give a handshake – being careful to get the grip right and not do it so tightly that they crush someone's hand. The same applies to being overly 'gushing' with the friends and family who didn't desert me – getting the balance right between expressing my gratitude and letting them know how much I love them, and over the top outpourings which make people feel uncomfortable. With this in mind, whilst some relationships didn't survive because of the damage that my alcoholism caused, my growing confidence enabled me to recognise some people who were not good for me. I realised that it suited those people for me to be a submissive alcoholic, and it would be unhealthy for me if they remained in my life.

I'm sharing this because I want you to know that no matter how far down the alcoholic spiral you have gone, you can get the old you back and more. My therapy session with Tim took me from a place of absolute despair and acceptance that I was going to die because I could never stop drinking, to a place where I was rebuilding my relationships with the people who genuinely loved me. I gained the self-respect and confidence to focus on those people and myself, and to recognise and 'let go' of the people who were not good for me. I was even beginning to like myself again.

And so eighteen months after I had spent the day with Tim, I found myself surrounded by the people I loved to celebrate Ross and my fiftieth birthdays, Michael's twenty first birthday and our tenth wedding anniversary, all rolled into one huge champagne fuelled party. I took a step back to look over the room, and I felt overwhelmed with gratitude. All the people who I loved and were important to me were there, including Mark and his wife. Tim had given me back everything that I had lost and so much more.

Chapter 10

Living A Happy, Sober Life Forever

As time passed and the enormity of what Tim had done for me became more apparent as my relationships continued to heal and confidence and optimism for the future increased, my compulsion to share the miracle of my survival with other alcoholics steadily grew stronger. The fact that thoughts of alcohol never even crossed my mind, even when I was with people who were drinking, completely blew me away because I had never expected the results of seeing Tim to be so profound.

As it became clear that this was my reality now and I knew that I would never drink alcohol again, I believed then, and still do, that it would be wrong of me to keep this to myself and simply get on with my life. My years of drinking had brought me into contact with so many desperate alcoholics who were trying so hard to stay sober and I wanted them to be given the same second chance that I had been given. I honestly wanted to shout it from the rooftops.

I became increasingly frustrated and then angry that the same old standard approaches for dealing with people with alcoholism have changed little for decades, and that the 'go to' option is still a Twelve Step programme, even though there is little evidence that this actually works long term. Even recovering alcoholics leaving rehab are often told that they should continue to attend regular AA meetings if they want to remain sober. It's as if AA is almost untouchable and anyone who dares challenge it is 'in denial', so they have ended up almost with a monopoly on alcoholism.

Because of my own experiences, I was also troubled about the amount of money some individuals and organisations make out of desperate and vulnerable alcoholics who will do, or pay, anything if they believe that it will help them to stop drinking. This includes rehabs which costs thousands of pounds and individuals like the hypnotherapists that I saw over the years who will still take money from an alcoholic, even when they know that they aren't adequately equipped to help someone with chronic alcoholism.

The more I realised how lucky I had been, the sadder I became about the number of hopeless alcoholics who would die because of inadequate treatment. As I said before, I have heard over time that some of the people I had met along the way in AA and rehab are now dead.

The problem was, and still is, that there is only one Tim and alcohol is not even his main focus - he deals with all kinds of serious issues from eating disorders to PTSD with his unique approach, which he has developed over years and years of helping people. But something else Tim does do is train other hypnotherapists. I knew that it would only need one trial using his approach to treat alcoholics in one health authority, to prove how successful his treatment is and then it could be rolled out across the NHS. The savings to the NHS would be immense, not only in terms of the treatment costs compared to counselling, CBT, rehab etc., but more importantly, the related cost burdens that alcohol problems place on the NHS, (illness, and accidents which fill up A&E etc.).

I decided that I had a compelling case and that I had to make people aware of this!

However while my enthusiasm and good intentions were commendable, I was probably naïve when I arranged an appointment relatively early in my sobriety with my local MP Chris Grayling at his constituency surgery, to explain my story and, hopefully, persuade him to get me in front of the Health Secretary.

It was most certainly too much too soon and, although he was very polite, he had much more pressing matters to attend to, (even though this was in the lead up to the Brexit referendum). For a long time after this, I decided that it was just better to keep my head down, focus on my relationships and earn some money, rather than trying to save the world.

And so, after the Chris Grayling episode, instead of going on a crusade to help others I did indeed keep my head down, focusing on making my life better and earning back the love and trust of Ross, Michael, my family and friends.

This was a good thing because over time, as the months since I had met Tim or had a drink of alcohol turned into a few years, my relationships began to heal and my confidence grew, I realised that my accrued years of sobriety gave me much more credibility to talk in a compelling way about my incredible transformation from hopeless alcoholic to survivor, which is when I decided to share my story.

Over time, I steadily equipped myself with some sensible tools to protect my sobriety, which are second nature to me now, and which I think could be very useful for others.

As I explained in Chapter 9, even though I know that I will never intentionally drink alcohol again, there is always a risk that this could happen accidentally and I never want alcohol to be allowed to enter my body in case it triggers some kind of chemical response that I then can't stop, (I don't even know if this is actually a scientific thing, I just want to avoid the risk completely). For this reason, I decided to never order alcohol free cocktails, in case a mistake is made by the person making it. When I was drinking, but attempting a period of sobriety, I would tell people that I was drinking an alcohol free cocktail, but would make sure that alcohol was added to it, or I would hope that the person behind the bar made a mistake and added alcohol, so I know from experience that alcohol free cocktails are a potential disaster for me.

In the same vein, I never drink alcohol free wine or beer. I just think, what's the point? I really don't want to risk the taste causing some trigger in my brain to click back into alcohol mode – I believe very strongly that when I met Tim it was a team effort and that I owe it to myself to avoid unnecessary risks because this would be foolish. I also never allow anyone that I do not know to pour my drinks, (at a party for example) and, if in doubt, I just don't drink it. My sobriety is so precious to me now because alcohol is basically my poison – my kryptonite.

On the odd occasion when I have inadvertently consumed alcohol in food, (Christmas mince pie, fish pie with hidden wine), I have been violently ill. This may well be psychological, (although I wasn't always aware that there might be alcohol in the food) but even if it is, I always check food labelling very thoroughly now, and I always say that I have an alcohol allergy in a restaurant in the same way that someone with a nut allergy does. I believe what Tim has done is 'hypnotic Antabuse', and I know now that even a tiny amount of alcohol can make me very ill.

Even though I avoid anything that could contain alcohol or which closely resembles it, I do like to drink out of an 'adult' glass when we are out or at a party, so that I don't feel different to other people. I also prefer to have drinks that I want to sip rather than gulp. It became apparent very quickly to me that the choices for someone who doesn't drink alcohol are very limited and can be quite boring, so I tend to drink the most fiery ginger beer that I can find, or a slim line tonic so that I can just sip them – and always from a wine glass.

I don't think this is so important to many people who choose not to drink alcohol, but there is something about being made to feel different, especially at an occasion like a wedding, when I'm not drinking from a flute for the Toast, that I can find awkward, even though I know that there will be people there who are driving and who won't be drinking champagne.

My friend Gayle's Mum was so kind to me at Gayle's wedding, when she asked the waiter to have my soft drink for the Toast put into a champagne flute, and I always stop the waiter from removing my wine glass in a restaurant, when they find out that I won't be drinking wine, and I then use it for my sparkling water - it's silly little things like that that can make a big difference to me.

In other areas of my life I have found many ways that I can help myself to make everyday life easier, after spending so many years drinking. One very important thing that I realised quickly is that many people have an entrenched perception of alcoholics and ex alcoholics and that is, 'once an alcoholic always an alcoholic'.

I understand that the majority of people will have little or no personal experience of alcoholism and so I didn't feel the need to tell everyone that I had been an alcoholic, especially when I re-entered the world of employment. There is still a huge stigma attached to alcoholism which is perpetuated by the belief in AA that you can never be 'cured', so I don't see any problem in someone who has had a drink problem keeping it to themselves when they want to.

Something else that I try to do frequently is to remind myself to 'forget regret or life is yours to miss'. I am and always will be acutely aware that I have wasted so much precious time and tragically lost a lot of my life to alcohol, and these are years and memories that I cannot ever get back. I consider it my 'self- inflicted dementia' and I try hard to focus on creating new memories instead of beating myself up over the ones I might have lost. Of course this doesn't always work and I do have moments of sorrow, guilt and regret because I am only human and the waste of time can be painful. However I try to be kind to myself and not let these feelings become overwhelming.

As I have become stronger over time, I have realised that negative emotions can be dangerous and corrosive, and they are the reason why my drinking took over my life in the first place, so I continue to actively try to remove negative things from my life. Even the smallest, most trivial changes can make a difference, from switching off depressing soap operas and miserable, exploitative programmes like Jeremy Kyle if I'm at home and have accidentally left the morning TV on in the background, to changing the password for my business accounts – I had been hacked a while ago and set my password to something about hating hackers. Then I realised that hate is such a negative word and that a more positive password about attracting success might actually have a beneficial effect. Silly, but you never know.

Negativity can also come from some of the people that we allow into our lives, and I have found that over time my sobriety has given me the confidence and strength to recognise if someone isn't good for my mental health, and then quietly and without fuss I surreptitiously remove these people from my life. I feel that I am making up for lost time, and I want to surround myself with people who make me a better person, not waste any more precious time with people who suck the energy out of a room or trigger negative thoughts or anxious feelings within me.

By the same token, I try not to allow myself to create negative feelings if at all possible, for example, I am determined never to tell lies because for years my whole life became one big lie. I believe that even white lies are, for me, pointless and damaging, so I try to be truthful and this makes my life so much simpler.

I do believe very strongly that my session with Tim was a team effort and that I owe it to myself to treat myself as a 'work in progress' and to continue to address aspects of my personality that I feel may let me down or hinder my happiness. Life for us all is constantly changing and throwing up new challenges and I, like everyone else, not just alcoholics, need to equip myself to handle difficult situations, and I accept that my years drinking 'stunted my growth' in this respect.

There have been so many difficult 'firsts' since I stopped drinking, like Ross facing the threat of redundancy, my own health scares and the sale of our house falling through multiple times which, in the past, would've made we want to drink.

Tim was kind enough to give me recordings which I now use frequently to remain positive, strong and motivated to make my life better and heal my relationships - to work on myself. For example, I used Tim's PSTEC recordings to help me to write this book because I have never done something like this before, and lacked the confidence to even know where to start. I am also prone to procrastination, basically finding any excuse to delay doing something because of my own fear of failure, but listening to Tim's recordings and tapping my fears away helped me keep going and built my confidence in writing down my experiences.

Dr Joe Dispenza's book, 'Breaking the Habit of Being Yourself' and his YouTube videos have also been especially helpful, (discovering him was one good thing that came out of my first rehab, Chapter 5). He explains very simply how our thoughts ultimately create our reality and so if we are having the same negative thoughts daily, we can't expect to create a happy and positive life for ourselves. I discovered that we can all 'create our day', and living in the most positive way I can is what I now aspire to, because my drinking life was so dark and negative.

Since I met Tim I have come to believe that we all have the power within us to 're-wire' our brain and completely change our lives and that there is so much truth in the philosophy –

"Watch your thoughts, they become words. Watch your words, they become actions. Watch your actions, they become habits. Watch your habits, they become your character. Watch your character, it becomes your destiny"

I also listen to and read about people who inspire me like Oprah Winfrey and I have always felt so empowered by a quote I found from Jamie Lee Curtis –

'I am more successful than I have ever been. I feel very positive where I never did before and I think that's all a direct result of getting sober'.

But although I constantly work on myself to help with the day to day challenges that we all face, I have never needed to revisit or work on my relationship with alcohol - there is no relationship with alcohol since I met Tim. As I have mentioned several times now, (but I do want to shout it from the rooftops), alcohol never even crosses my mind, ever since I left Tim's office, and so I never need to spend any time reminding myself of what is was like, or how bad things became.

It is interesting, however, that I do very occasionally have 'drinking dreams', which many people talked about in AA. During these dreams I completely fall of the wagon and they are so real and disturbing that for the first few seconds when I wake up, I actually believe that I have let everyone down, experiencing all of the extreme fear, panic and anxiety that comes with that belief. I have read that these dreams are very common for people who used to drink and they are a very powerful reminder for me of feelings that I never want to experience in real life again.

Another thing that was talked about a lot in AA, is how many relationships don't survive after a person gets sober. The confidence that they regain and the reassessment of their lives that they naturally go through, can sometimes highlight flaws in close relationships that they were never aware of before because they were drunk.

I am so blessed and feel incredibly lucky that the two most important people, Ross and Michael, are still in my life and I will spend my lifetime making it up to them. I couldn't have written this book without their blessing and support, which they have so generously given me, even though it brings back very painful memories that they would rather forget, and has revealed new details about that secret life that I had hidden from them, which I know has been upsetting.

I mentioned in Chapter 9 that I made a decision early on not to rush myself or anyone around me, or expect too much from them, but that doesn't mean that healing my relationships wasn't at the top of my list of priorities. It's a huge testament to Ross and Michael that they have believed in me and trusted me, never once using my alcoholism as a weapon or bringing it up in a hurtful manner, even though it impacted on their lives in such a destructive way. And this is also true of my family and closest friends.

I mention this because I know that other alcoholics may not be so lucky, but no one close to me has ever used my drinking in a cruel way or made fun of me about it, even though I did some very hurtful and embarrassing things. If someone had cancer in the past or had completely recovered from a stroke, people around them wouldn't keep reminding them of 'the bad old days' and I don't see why alcoholism should be any different. Of course I am more than happy to talk about it, otherwise I would not be writing this book, but I wouldn't expect anyone to make fun of me about it or talk about it with the intention of making me feel ashamed.

So in terms of my relationships, I have made 'fixing' them my priority and, although I now have a much smaller circle of close friends, these are the ones that make me a better person, my 'two o clock in the morning' friends, who I know I could phone at any time and they would be there for me. I try hard to 'nurture' these friendships like you would a plant that you love, as I do with my family. I let them down so often before, that I now make sure that I reply to messages immediately, arrange dates to see them frequently and basically let them know how much they mean to me.

Second nature to most, but these were things that I let slip for years.

There are friends that I lost because I was drinking and some that are no longer in my life because I stopped drinking and this reminds me of something else important that I have learned. You will absolutely need to make amends with some people if you have been an alcoholic, because you can't live your life in such chaos and self-destruction without doing or saying some awful things that you will need to say sorry for, but good friends will not expect you to eat humble pie forever.

Finally, I have learned that in a healthy friendship we are equal and the 'nurturing' should be a two-way thing, and being sober has again given me the confidence over time to recognise if a friendship has become one way traffic. Again this is just basic stuff for most people, but something that I have had to re-learn.

And so with time and the love and support of Ross and Michael and my friends and family, I have reached a stage where I feel like I have earned the right to 'shout it from the rooftops' like I wanted to do a few years ago when I went to see my local MP.

I firmly believe, as do those around me who saw me at my worst, that what Tim has done for me is nothing short of a miracle, but it is a miracle that could so easily be made available for other alcoholics who desperately want to get sober, and that doesn't just mean people who have got to the absolute end of the line like me, but anyone who knows that they are on the alcoholic spiral.

I worry that, as a society, we are sleepwalking towards an alcohol-induced disaster, and that our current drinking habits– especially among ordinary women like me– are a ticking time bomb. I believe that increasing numbers of people like me will become ill, wreck their lives and die young, because drinking excessive amounts of alcohol is steadily being normalised. Our current drinking habits already place a burden on the NHS, (liver disease, which used to be seen mainly in elderly men, is on the increase in younger women, for example), and this is only going to get worse and, ultimately, children and grandchildren are going to be left without parents and grandparents. For so many people I have met, drinking dangerous amounts of alcohol is not only acceptable, but encouraged. Wine o'clock and gin o'clock are innocently referred to on social media with a giggle.

I know from experience that not all excessive drinkers will become alcoholics – there are many, varied factors that create a problem drinker – but our society's casual attitude towards excessive drinking and getting wasted can only increase the numbers of people developing alcoholism in the future. How often have you seen stories in the news about someone disrupting a flight when they are so intoxicated that they turn violent or abusive because they have been refused more alcohol, or stories about ordinary men and women causing injury and death on the roads because they are over the limit?

And that brings me on to alcohol itself. As I said in Chapter 3, when I came out of my second rehab, I noticed almost for the first time that alcohol is absolutely everywhere, which makes it extremely difficult for someone who is trying to stay sober. Unlike someone who is, for example, trying to stay clean after being addicted to a Class A drug, alcohol is socially acceptable, so a recovering alcoholic will have to deal not only with seeing alcohol everywhere (on TV, in shops, the homes of friends, in cooking recipes) but they will probably sometimes be around people who are heavily under the influence.

As my friend in AA who had many years of sobriety behind her once told me, being around people drinking made the alcoholic inside her, her dark shadow, 'stir' and I am lucky not to have that problem - mine has gone forever.

I heard many times in rehab and AA that if alcohol was invented now, it too would be a Class A drug, because of its addictive properties, the harm that it does and the impact that it has on our health and society in general. However, since alcohol has become so embedded in our culture and socially acceptable to drink, it would now be extremely difficult to change how we classify alcohol and the laws relating to it and, because of that, there will always be alcoholics.

So how do you know that you are an alcoholic, or if someone that you love or care about is an alcoholic? The conclusion that I have come to over the years, which has come from my personal experience and what I have learned and observed form people that I have met, is that it is most certainly not how much you drink or what you drink, but the motivation behind your drinking that distinguishes an alcoholic from someone who simply likes a drink - even heavy drinkers may not be alcoholics.

If a person always drinks with the intention of getting drunk, this should ring alarm bells and I know that once I started to drink, I always wanted to get drunk. More obviously, if drinking always has a detrimental effect on your time with others or is having a negative impact on your life, yet you still cannot or won't stop, or you can't even see that there is a connection between problems in your life and drinking, then you have an unhealthy relationship with alcohol.

I used to turn any situation into an excuse to drink and it was always the drinking aspect of a social event that I fixated on, for example, the pint after a long country walk, the champagne at a celebration, the mulled wine at a Christmas carol service, wine during a romantic meal….. It got to the point where the actual occasion and the people I was meant to be enjoying it with weren't important anymore. I might as well have been at home alone. More apparent warning signs are obviously lying about how much you've been drinking, hiding it, and getting defensive or aggressive if it is mentioned.

Finally, and even though this seems obvious it is not always obvious to an alcoholic, I believe that anyone who drinks and then drives needs to question why they cannot resist having a drink when they know that they are going to get behind the wheel.

I decided that I had to share my own experiences because I know that there are so many people these days who are worried about their own drinking or how much someone they love is drinking and I also know how frightening it is when you just can't stop, even when you have tried time and time again to get sober.

The treatment options available to most alcoholics are the same as they have been for years and are woefully inadequate. If another illness caused the amount of death, suffering and damage to society that alcoholism does there would be a public outcry and resources would be found to research alternative treatments. The horrible three out of ten statistic that I was made aware of in rehab would not be tolerated.

I know that there will be people who read my book and come to the conclusion that I had not reached rock bottom when I went to rehab or spent time in the rooms of AA and that is why I started to drink again. I think that my notes to Ross and Michael begging for forgiveness and another chance are proof that I wanted to get sober more than anything and I know how terrified realising I was an alcoholic made me feel. I did not want to live, or die, that way.

If I was allowed to go into AA meetings with a 'captive audience' of alcoholics to talk to about my escape from alcoholism, that would be a start, but I know that I would not be welcome there because they would have a problem with the fact that I know that I will never drink again and I am not living sober 'one day at a time'. It is frustrating because I want other alcoholics to have what I now have - the absolute freedom to enjoy any experience with their loved ones without having to avoid their own triggers, (places, people, events), or to feel the need to place constraints on what their friends and family can do around them. Parties, Christmas, weddings, holidays, meals out, romantic nights in - to be able to share all of these with people who are drinking, without experiencing the draining inner battle of trying to resist alcohol, or the energy sapping torture of mustering up as much willpower as possible to stop yourself from being tempted to drink.

Tim uses his approach to help people with many issues, from eating disorders to PTSD and he is so confident in its success that he has basically thrown down the gauntlet to test his methods against the 'go to' treatments available on the NHS, and he has put out a Media Challenge –

'I created my Media Challenge simply because there's an important point which needs addressing. Many people tell me that they've undergone common NHS treatments such as CBT or counselling and gotten nowhere. To prove that better methods genuinely do exist I created my national media challenge .... Pitch me on TV or Radio directly against any NHS therapist, counsellor, psychologist, psychiatrist, (or other large and well known mental health institution); using NHS approved therapies for any of the kinds of issues listed on this page. I'll publicly demonstrate that my own methods are many times better than theirs and much faster too.'

I needed to write my book mainly because I want to help people who find themselves in the desperate and bleak place that I found myself in, and I believe that I have a duty to share my story because it could help so many others – I feel it would be selfish of me not to do so. But there is another very important reason for my book, and this is to try to get the powers that be to take notice and explore alternative treatments. Maybe even to take Tim up on his Media Challenge, so that he can train more people to do the amazing work that he does with people who so desperately need help.
When you consider the huge costs of rehab or a lifelong commitment to AA, as well as the money spent by the NHS on drinking related illnesses and people ending up in A and E because of alcohol, it seems crazy to me that Tim hasn't been given the opportunity to train a small army of people, or even just given the opportunity to carry out a small trial within the NHS. Saving lives and saving money. Hopefully if nothing else, sharing my story will at least raise awareness of what Tim does.

However I want to end here with my most important message, and that is for the poor alcoholics reading this book who are feeling isolated and alone.

I know that you are desperate and think that there is no hope, but the very fact that you are reading this shows that you still want to help yourself. I know that you have a massive amount of love inside you for your family and friends and you can still tap into this to help you overcome your seemingly impossible situation. There will also be so much love around you, from which you can draw strength, even if you think that people have given up on you. I understand exactly how you are feeling, but I can also promise you that no matter how wretched you are and how hopeless things seem, life can get better and you can beat this – and being sober is not as scary as I know that you imagine it will be. People who love you really will be kind and they will forgive you. You can laugh again and dance again and the only dark shadow you will have, will be your own shadow in the bright sunshine.

So do it now. Make a resolution and commitment to giving yourself another chance. You really do deserve that. You can beat this. And, most importantly - never, ever, ever give up.

Present Day

Michael is happy, successful and following his dreams in Law and we are closer than ever.

Me and Ross are very happy and laugh a lot - life is never boring in a good way.

My niece Jenny trusts me to babysit.

Mark is very happily married

Tim Phizackerley britainsfastesthypnotist.com

Tim's approach has been evolved into an App called Orpheus, for anyone who wants to cut down or control their drinking.

www.orpheusmindtechnologies.com

Contact me anytime at –

Susan Laurie susan@soberforever.co.uk

Printed in Great Britain
by Amazon

43842703R00116